CASE FORMULATION
WITH CHILDREN AND ADOLESCENTS

Also from Katharina Manassis

*Problem Solving in Child and Adolescent Psychotherapy:
A Skills-Based, Collaborative Approach*

Case Formulation with Children and Adolescents

KATHARINA MANASSIS

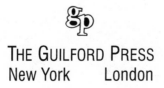

THE GUILFORD PRESS
New York   London

Printed in the United States of America

This book is printed on acid-free paper.

Last digit is print number: 9 8 7 6 5 4 3 2

The author has checked with sources believed to be reliable in her efforts to provide information that is complete and generally in accord with the standards of practice that are accepted
at the time of publication. However, in view of the possibility of human error or changes in
behavioral, mental health, or medical sciences, neither the author, nor the editor and pub-
lisher, nor any other party who has been involved in the preparation or publication of this
work warrants that the information contained herein is in every respect accurate or complete,
and they are not responsible for any errors or omissions or the results obtained from the use
of such information. Readers are encouraged to confirm the information contained in this
book with other sources.

Library of Congress Cataloging-in-Publication Data

Manassis, Katharina, author.
  Case formulation with children and adolescents / by Katharina Manassis.
    pages cm
  Includes bibliographical references and index.
  ISBN 978-1-4625-1560-8 (hardback : acid-free paper)
  1. Psychiatry—Case formulation.   2. Interviewing in child psychiatry.
  3. Interviewing in adolescent psychiatry.   4. Child psychiatry—Differential
therapeutics.   I. Title.
  RC473.C37M36 2014
  616.89—dc23
                                                                    2014003703

About the Author

Katharina Manassis, MD, FRCPC, is Staff Psychiatrist and Senior Associate Scientist at the Hospital for Sick Children in Toronto, where she established and continues to work in the Anxiety Disorders Program for children and youth. The program focuses on the development and scientific evaluation of cognitive-behavioral treatments. Dr. Manassis is also Professor in the Department of Psychiatry at the University of Toronto and a member of the Human Development and Applied Psychology Department at the Ontario Institute for Studies in Education. These appointments allow her to supervise graduate students, residents, and fellows in the treatment and study of childhood anxiety. Dr. Manassis leads several funded research studies to better understand and treat childhood anxiety disorders. She is the author of more than 70 papers in professional journals in this field and of two widely read books for parents, *Keys to Parenting Your Anxious Child* and *Helping Your Teenager Beat Depression*, as well as books for child mental health professionals, including *Problem Solving in Child and Adolescent Psychotherapy*.

Introduction

When I began my training in child and adolescent psychiatry in the 1980s, one of the first skills I was required to learn was case formulation. That is, after interviewing a child or adolescent and his or her family, I was expected to present to my supervisor a coherent story of how this young person's difficulties had come about. Then, based on this story, I had to propose treatment(s) that would be helpful in ameliorating those difficulties. The starting point for the story was a table listing various biological, psychological, and social factors that might be contributing to the youth's problems. I soon learned that the same table of factors could be synthesized into multiple different stories, depending on the interests and theoretical orientation of the supervisor. In fact, clever and ambitious trainees would tailor the case formulation to a supervisor's preferences. Occasionally, I encountered a supervisor who emphasized diagnosis over case formulation, but most supervisors at that time dismissed diagnosis as "mere phenomenology" and believed strongly in case formulation.

Over the years, discoveries in neuroscience and child development have profoundly altered the nature of the factors used in case formulation with children and adolescents. Clinicians have also increasingly recognized the importance of cultural and spiritual factors in addition to biological, psychological, and social ones. Although these developments have significantly changed the content of most case formulations, the process of case formulation has not changed nearly as much.

Clinicians must still carefully gather information from children, families, teachers, and other professionals, and then synthesize the information into a coherent story, use the story to inform treatment, and communicate the story effectively to all concerned.

Revision of the case formulation in response to new information, however, has received greater emphasis in recent years. The case formulation is no longer seen as a definitive, unchanging explanation of psychopathology but rather a hypothesis to be tested and modified over time. This change makes sense, as mental health professionals on the whole now take a more empirical approach to their work than they did in the past. In other words, they are willing to concede that if a youth's behavior is inconsistent with their initial hypothesis, then maybe the hypothesis was incorrect.

In addition, most mental health professionals no longer see diagnosis and case formulation as competitors. Instead, these two approaches are seen as complementary, with each offering helpful perspectives on the young person's distress and therapeutic needs. Recently, the case formulation approach has enjoyed renewed interest as clinicians have appreciated the limits of relying solely on diagnostic categories. For example, the dimensional approach to psychopathology in DSM-5 may reflect the recognition that people present with complex mental health issues that are not always amenable to neat categorization. Of course, some classification of psychopathology is still important if we are to communicate effectively about mental health and mental illness, but when a young person doesn't fit a particular category, it is important to seek a more nuanced understanding of his or her symptoms.

Recent advances in child development and public education about mental health have also renewed interest in case formulation. Developmental psychopathologists are increasingly able to elucidate the complex interplay between various risk and protective factors and between various genetic and environmental effects. As a result, our efforts to formulate children's difficulties are becoming less speculative and increasingly rooted in developmental science. Moreover, as families are becoming more educated about their children's mental health, they expect clinicians to provide a holistic, developmentally sophisticated understanding of their children in addition to an accurate diagnosis. In short, the case formulation appears to be an old idea whose time has come again.

On a practical level, the case formulation enhances mental health care for children and adolescents. It is a systematic approach, reducing the chances of missing key pieces of information relevant to a case. Case formulation can provide helpful, parsimonious explanatory models for children with complex comorbid conditions or for children who do not resemble typical subjects studied in treatment-focused research. Children who fail to respond to evidence-based treatment or are wait-listed for treatment may also benefit from a case formulation, particularly when attention is paid to factors that may perpetuate their symptoms. Furthermore, as the case formulation process yields testable hypotheses about each youth's difficulties, it encourages careful monitoring and an empirical approach to evaluating his or her progress with treatment.

Unfortunately, case formulation is neither easy to learn nor easy to teach to clinicians new to child and adolescent work. The task of weaving together knowledge of children's psychological development (typical and pathological), with an understanding of common childhood disorders, temperament and genetic influences, parenting and family life, academics and school life, and the multitude of cultural and social influences in children's lives today is difficult. Assessment involving multiple informants (i.e., parents, teachers, and other professionals, as well as the child or adolescent) poses the further challenges of synthesizing information that may be inconsistent or contradictory and of communicating findings in a way that is sensitive and helpful to all parties. It is, therefore, surprising that a book dedicated to understanding case formulation with children and adolescents does not already exist. This book is intended to fill that unfortunate gap.

Based on my experience as a child psychiatrist, I wrote this book to highlight elements of the case formulation that I consider important or that are easily overlooked, which can result in adverse consequences for the young person. First, important aspects of child and adolescent assessment and of each of the contributing factors (biological, psychological, social, and spiritual–cultural) are reviewed in the context of child development. Then, the challenges of case formulation particular to each age group (preschoolers, school-age children, adolescents) are illustrated with detailed case examples. Last, the skills required to communicate the case formulation effectively, to use it to best inform treatment, and to revise it when necessary are described.

My principal reason for writing this book, however, is to convey some of the joy of seeking to understand the world of a child or adolescent. Intellectually, the case formulation process is similar to solving an intricate puzzle. However, unlike solving a crossword or Sudoku puzzle, finding the solution to a case formulation puzzle can actually make a difference in someone's life, making it a more satisfying and meaningful pursuit. What a privilege! Friends sometimes ask me if my work gets boring or if I've "seen it all" after a quarter century in practice. My honest reply is that every case formulation, every attempt to understand and to identify a young person's strengths as well as difficulties, is an adventure. Case formulation reminds me that each child and adolescent I meet and care for is unique, and uniquely interesting after all these years.

Contents

Purchasers may download larger versions of selected figures from
www.guilford.com/manassis2-forms.

CHAPTER 1

Benefits of Case Formulation and a Conceptual Framework

THE CASE OF MALCOLM

Malcolm's third-grade teacher noticed that he seemed unfocused. He was frequently caught off guard when asked a question, and he rarely finished assigned tasks. The teacher suggested to Malcolm's parents that they investigate the possibility that Malcolm had attention-deficit/hyperactivity disorder (ADHD). Malcolm's mother indicated that she had not found Malcolm to be inattentive at home, and added immediately, "And I will not have my child drugged because you don't know how to teach him." She acknowledged, however, that her son sometimes had stomachaches before school and thought that his family doctor should refer Malcolm for a mental health assessment to determine if he had an anxiety disorder. Malcolm's father, on the other hand, stated, "The boy is fine. He's a little lazy sometimes, but that's because his mother is too soft with him." Nobody asked Malcolm about his difficulties.

After his mother spoke to the family doctor, Malcolm was referred to a child mental health clinic for an anxiety-focused assessment. The psychiatry resident in the clinic did a thorough diagnostic interview with Malcolm's mother, briefly evaluated Malcolm's mental status, and concluded that Malcolm met criteria for ADHD, inattentive type, and generalized anxiety disorder. Given his mother's aversion to using stimulant medication (the evidence-based treatment of choice

1

for ADHD), the resident referred Malcolm for anxiety-focused, group-based cognitive-behavioral therapy (CBT), a therapy focused on changing anxious thoughts and behaviors).

The group therapist noticed that Malcolm seemed unfocused, was often caught off guard when asked a question, and rarely finished assigned tasks. She asked for a meeting with Malcolm's parents in order to explain to them that he was deriving little benefit from the group, and they should consider having him treated for his primary diagnosis (ADHD). Malcolm's mother responded with a voice mail message indicating that she and her husband had recently separated, so he would not be attending the meeting. At the meeting, she reiterated her opposition to medication and declined further mental health treatment for Malcolm. She told the therapist that she was planning to enroll Malcolm in a private school "once his father starts paying child support."

Malcolm's parents became embroiled in a bitter custody battle that lasted 3 years. During this time, Malcolm's school performance continued to deteriorate.

WHAT WENT WRONG IN THIS CASE?

At first glance, it seems that Malcolm is merely the victim of unfortunate circumstances. His teacher correctly identified his difficulty focusing, resulting in an eventual diagnosis of ADHD. His family doctor referred him to a mental health clinic that was able to provide a thorough diagnostic assessment. The assessment confirmed that the observations of Malcolm's teacher and his mother were correct, and he indeed had two diagnoses: ADHD and generalized anxiety disorder. The treatments recommended (stimulant medication for ADHD and CBT for the anxiety disorder) were both evidence based and appropriate. One could perhaps argue that Malcolm would have derived more benefit from individual rather than group-based psychotherapy, but given the large number of children who need mental health services, individual therapy is not always readily available.

Malcolm's poor outcome, however, begs the question "What else could the mental health professionals involved have done in this case?" Should they have obtained more details about the relationships within Malcolm's family, rather than focusing exclusively on diagnostic criteria during the assessment? Should they have explored the possibility that Malcolm might have a learning disability, seizure disorder, or other neurological reason for his inattention? Would they have learned more if they spent more time interviewing Malcolm? Would it have been worthwhile to explore the reasons why Malcolm's mother was so opposed to medication?

A cynic might reply, "Hindsight is 20/20. They did the best they could, given what they knew at the time." While there is some truth to this statement, it is also rather discouraging. In my practice as a child psychiatrist and child psychiatric consultant, I have run across far too many children with histories that are similar to Malcolm's story. Professionals involved in these cases are often knowledgeable and well intentioned and meet the minimum standard of practice. Regrettably, they miss key pieces of relevant information when assessing these children, often with disastrous results.

THE GOAL OF THIS BOOK

The main goal of this book is to reduce the number of "Malcolm stories" in the field of children's mental health. To achieve this goal, a case formulation approach is presented that illustrates how to systematically collect and synthesize information that is relevant to understanding presenting problems in child mental health. The case formulation approach is not specific to any one discipline but can inform the practice of all professionals who evaluate and treat children with mental health difficulties.

Information used in case formulation includes symptoms relevant to diagnosis as well as historical and contextual information that provides a more complete understanding of the child's life and his or her emotional and behavioral problems. The latter information not only provides an enhanced understanding of the child but is also very useful clinically. Synthesized effectively, such information allows clinicians to generate linked hypotheses about why a particular child presents with particular difficulties. This set of linked hypotheses constitutes the case formulation. When defining case formulation, experts in the field have emphasized three important elements: 1) the case formulation as hypotheses about factors contributing to a person's emotional and behavioral problems; 2) the case formulation as a means of organizing complex and sometimes contradictory information about a person's difficulties; 3) the case formulation as a blueprint for guiding treatment (Eells, 2006, p. 4). Case formulation hypotheses can be tested and (if needed) revised as the child develops and responds or fails to respond to treatment. Thus, the child's response provides evidence that either supports or fails to support certain hypotheses, allowing a more and more accurate case formulation to emerge over time.

Before describing case formulation in more detail, however, it is important to dispel two common misconceptions and to provide a conceptual framework that will be used in this book. The two misconceptions are (1) that people who practice case formulation do not value mental health diagnoses, and (2) that the process of case formulation is unscientific or not evidence based. Each of these misconceptions is now discussed, followed by a description of key concepts used throughout this book.

DIAGNOSIS AND CASE FORMULATION

The title of this section, "diagnosis *and* case formulation," reflects the idea that these two approaches do not compete with but rather complement each other. Each has something different to offer, as shown in Table 1.1. Diagnosis in children's mental health, whether described in the *Diagnostic and Statistical Manual of Mental Disorders* (DSM-5; American Psychiatric Association, 2013) or the *International Classification of Diseases* (ICD-10; World Health Organization, 1994), is based on phenomenology. That is, it is based on the presence or absence of certain symptoms or behaviors in the child. For many diagnoses, the symptoms must be present for a certain length of time and/or interfere with the child's day-to-day functioning. In many jurisdictions, the privilege of assigning a diagnosis is restricted to certain child mental health professionals, typically psychiatrists and psychologists.

The child mental health diagnosis does not, however, imply any particular cause for the child's symptoms. In theory, this ensures that the diagnosis is based on objective facts, rather than being subject to the clinician's (often subjective) speculations about causality. In practice, diagnostic information about young children is often obtained from adults around the child, and is thus influenced by the objectivity (or lack thereof) of the observer. Nevertheless, diagnostic information is considered relatively objective and provides a helpful shorthand for professional communication. Saying, "This adolescent suffers from bipolar affective disorder," for example, is clearer and faster than listing all of the adolescent's symptoms that may relate to this diagnosis. Assigning a diagnosis can also be helpful when seeking access to resources for a particular child. For example, in the school system,

TABLE 1.1. Comparing Diagnostic and Case Formulation Approaches

Diagnostic approach	Case formulation approach
Based on phenomenology (symptoms)	Includes ideas about etiology as well as phenomenology
Restricted to psychiatrists and psychologists	Not restricted by discipline
Less speculative	More speculative
Easy to communicate	More difficult to communicate
Can be used to access resources	Not helpful in accessing resources
More stigmatizing	Less stigmatizing
Sometimes results in "lumping" dissimilar children	Treats each child and his or her difficulties as unique
More likely to result in missing relevant contextual or historical information	Less likely to result in missing relevant contextual or historical information
Sometimes results in erroneous assumptions about etiology	Results in testable hypotheses about etiology

children who are diagnosed as being on the autism spectrum and suffer from learning disabilities often have access to more educational supports than children with learning disabilities who do not have this diagnosis.

Disadvantages of diagnosis include stigmatization, an overly narrow understanding of the child's difficulties, and the potential for erroneous assumptions about causality and about different children who meet criteria for the same diagnosis. Stigmatization occurs when the diagnostic label is considered shameful by the child, family, or others. In some cultures, any mental health diagnosis is considered stigmatizing. In other cultures, only some mental health conditions (e.g., addictions or schizophrenia) are considered stigmatizing. Public education efforts in recent years have tried to ameliorate mental health stigma in North America, but some prejudice toward people with certain mental health problems remains. On the other hand, when children are already stigmatized by certain behaviors (e.g., a child with unusual rituals or tics who stands out in class), providing a diagnostic label (such as obsessive–compulsive disorder or Tourette syndrome) may help explain the behaviors to others and thus serve to reduce stigma.

Malcolm's story, just described, illustrates the pitfalls of an overly narrow understanding of the child's difficulties, in particular an understanding based almost exclusively on diagnostic information. Some clinicians make treatment decisions based on the assumption that a particular diagnosis implies a particular etiology. In Malcolm's case, the psychiatry resident assumed that his diagnosis of ADHD, inattentive type, implied a need for stimulant medication without considering the possibility of an underlying learning disability, distraction related to emotional distress (given the high-conflict home environment), or other reason for his inattention. The decision to refer Malcolm to the anxiety-focused cognitive-behavioral group was based on the diagnosis of generalized anxiety disorder, and the assumption that children with this diagnosis are all similar enough to benefit from the same treatment. In Malcolm's case, this assumption was false.

Case formulation, by contrast, includes a wider range of information than diagnosis does and thus has the potential to lead to a broader, more complete understanding of the child's difficulties. Case formulation assumes that each child has unique reasons for presenting with his or her difficulties, reducing the potential for erroneously "lumping" dissimilar children into the same category. In Malcolm's case, a clinician using a case formulation approach would have gathered additional information about his home environment, his early development (both medical and psychological aspects), and his previous learning history. His relationships with each of his parents, with his teacher, and with his peer group would also have been explored from multiple points of view (Malcolm and his parents at a minimum; ideally his teacher as well). Gathering such information is described in more detail in the next chapter.

Synthesizing this information to create a case formulation is, of necessity, more speculative than assigning a diagnosis. Case formulation includes examining various contributing factors and possible causes for the child's difficulties, as well as a detailed description of symptoms. Most practitioners, however, are careful to phrase their ideas as *possibilities*, rather than certainties. In addition, because the case formulation contains testable hypotheses, it lends itself to objective evaluation over time. Essentially, the various interventions and the child's response or lack of response to them become an experiment that allows the clinician to identify the most valid aspects of the formulation and the aspects requiring refinement. Thus, case formulation has the potential to complement diagnosis in order to determine the most effective intervention(s) for a given child.

Case formulation is sometimes less stigmatizing than diagnosis, but not always. Some parents, for example, feel stigmatized when clinicians explore family interactions or past childrearing practices in relation to the child's symptoms. Also, case formulation cannot generally be used to advocate for additional resources for children, and communicating a case formulation to another professional is usually more time-consuming than communicating a diagnosis.

In summary, diagnosis and case formulation both make unique contributions to the evaluation of mental health problems in children. Therefore, they should not be seen as competing approaches. Most children benefit from mental health assessments that include both.

EVIDENCE-BASED PRACTICE AND CASE FORMULATION

The idea that case formulation is incompatible with evidence-based practice is a myth. Usually, this myth is based on a false understanding of what constitutes evidence-based practice, a false understanding of how to use case formulation, or both.

When describing evidence-based practice, experts usually emphasize that it includes but is not limited to research findings. For example, in a well-known evidence-based practice model, Parry, Roth, and Fonagy (2005) suggest that evidence-based practice adhere to clinical practice guidelines that are based on both research findings and expert consensus. These guidelines should be applied using clinical judgment that is based on a clear formulation of the patient's difficulties (Parry et al., 2005). Thus, these authors see case formulation as an important component of evidence-based practice.

Moreover, basing one's practice exclusively on research findings could be problematic, due to the many limitations of existing research in child mental health and the unique nature of each child. Some important research limitations to bear in mind include the tendency for researchers to focus on interventions that are easy to study (Roth & Fonagy, 2005); the differences between success in academic practice (called "efficacy") and success in community practice (called "effectiveness") (Manassis, 2009a); differences in outcomes depending on who is reporting outcome (Kazdin, 1994); frequent lack of attention to child functioning and to long-term follow-up (Adler-Nevo & Manassis, 2009); and the absence of high-quality studies for some conditions (e.g., see Manassis, 2009b, regarding selective mutism). For example, CBT is easier to study than many other psychotherapies because it is time limited (allowing the researcher to finish his or her study in a short, defined granting period) and well described in specific manuals (making it relatively easy to measure therapist adherence and to replicate studies in different sites). These research advantages may amplify the number of positive studies for CBT relative to other therapies. Differences between the concepts of efficacy and effectiveness may result in disappointment in clinical practice, as interventions that work in research settings are often not nearly as helpful in community practice. Reasons for this phenomenon include more disadvantaged populations and more complex presentations in community settings, frequent lack of training or lack of supervision of community practitioners, and practice parameters that differ from those of academic centers (e.g., lack of diagnostic interviews prior to treatment, limited number of treatment sessions permitted). Research findings also need to be interpreted carefully with respect to informant, as children and parents often provide different reports of outcome (Barbosa, Manassis, & Tannock, 2002). One must also question the clinical meaning of studies that report improvement in symptoms but do not comment on the child's overall functioning or report improvement immediately posttreatment but do not provide follow-up data. Finally, it can be difficult to find reliable data on some child mental health conditions. For example, there are very few randomized controlled trials regarding the treatment of selective mutism (a condition where children do not speak in certain social environments), and most of the literature consists of case reports (Manassis, 2009b).

A further problem with relying exclusively on research findings when planning treatment occurs when clinicians try to fit children into particular diagnostic categories that have been studied. As we discussed, diagnosis is not a problem per se, but few children in community practice fit neatly into a single diagnostic category. Comorbidity (the occurrence of more than one psychiatric condition) is very high in child mental health, and the presence of one disorder may affect the treatment of another. For example, in the case described earlier, Malcolm's ADHD affected his ability to learn anxiety management skills in CBT. Even in the absence of comorbidity, children with the same diagnosis do not all respond to a given treatment in the same way. Research studies usually describe *average* degrees of change in response to treatment for dozens, sometimes hundreds of children. Therefore, if two children have the same diagnosis and receive the same treatment, they will not necessarily show equal benefit. Some studies describe moderators of outcome (factors associated with better or worse outcomes), but it is still not possible to precisely predict treatment response for an individual child.

Therefore, to best serve individual children, astute clinicians think about how the children they treat resemble or differ from those studied in relevant research, consult clinical practice guidelines, and apply their knowledge in the context of a clear, thoughtful case formulation (see Figure 1.1). In devising the formulation, clinicians synthesize information about biological, psychological, social, and spiritual influences on the child and their interactions. The formulation is not, however, a static, rigid set of beliefs or causal attributions. Rather, it is a dynamic set of hypotheses that provide one possible explanation for the child's difficulties (the "explanatory model"), which can be tested and revised. Treatment response or lack of response tests the hypotheses, supporting or disconfirming them. Hypotheses are then updated to create a revised formulation that is consistent with this new information. Additional information, life events or other changes in the child's environment, and developmental changes (including those resulting from the child's response to treatment) can also result in the need for an updated, revised formulation. Ongoing revision of the formulation allows for a better understanding of the child over time and improves the chances of providing ever more effective care. When an accurate

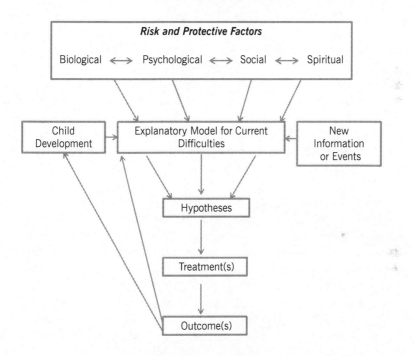

FIGURE 1.1. The dynamic case formulation.

formulation is shared with the child and family, feeling understood in turn can improve their motivation to work with the practitioner, contributing to further progress.

In summary, when used appropriately, case formulation supports and often enhances evidence-based practice by allowing clinicians to apply both research evidence and case-specific information to develop an effective plan of care for each individual child.

A CONCEPTUAL FRAMEWORK FOR CASE FORMULATION IN CHILD MENTAL HEALTH

Since first described by George Engel (1977), the biopsychosocial approach to case formulation has been widely used in medicine and mental health care. Rather than merely focusing on a particular disease process, this model advocates examining a variety of biological, psychological, and social factors that might be contributing to the patient's presentation. Interactions among these factors are also considered. Thus, the model takes a more holistic and humanistic approach to care than the disease-focused approach. In the last decade or so, many authors have advocated expanding this model to one that is biopsychosocial–spiritual (Skinner, 2009). Originally, the addition of spiritual considerations was advocated when treating addictions (in 12-step programs) or when treating the grieving or dying patient, but recently it has become a part of many general medical and mental health curricula as well. When clinicians work with people from cultural backgrounds that differ from their own, sensitivity to diverse beliefs, values, and spiritual practices is particularly relevant, so the final dimension of the model is sometimes defined broadly as "spiritual/cultural considerations."

In child mental health, the biopsychosocial–spiritual model needs to be understood in the context of children's ongoing development. The same problem may have a completely different meaning in an older child than in a younger child, and be due to different biological, psychological, social, and spiritual factors. A 4-year-old who has not previously attended day care and is anxious about leaving the house to start kindergarten, for example, may not be considered abnormal. His difficulty is probably due to a somewhat inhibited temperament (biological factor), a family environment that limited opportunities to spend time away from home (social factor), and parental values or beliefs (spiritual/cultural factor), with the result being a lack of confidence about his own ability to cope with unfamiliar environments (psychological factor). By contrast, a 14-year-old who suddenly develops a fear of leaving the house to go to school requires a thorough mental health assessment. There could be numerous factors contributing to this presentation, and the sudden onset of symptoms suggests that a significant stress or trauma has recently occurred.

To better understand how various biological, psychological, social, and spiritual factors interact throughout development, the field of developmental psychopathology has grown increasingly salient. This field has been defined as "an integrative discipline that seeks to unify, within a developmental, lifespan framework, contributions from multiple fields of inquiry with the goal of understanding psychopathology and its relation to normative adaptation" (Cicchetti, 1990, p. 3). Because it is defined as an "integrative discipline," developmental psychopathology can include various theories and ideas, and thus serve as a framework for discussions of children's cognitive, emotional, and behavioral development. This framework is used throughout the book as various aspects of case formulation are examined.

Developmental psychopathologists have enriched our understanding of children's risk factors as well as sources of resilience for various disorders. They are interested in developmental pathways as well as outcomes. The pathway that an individual follows for a given characteristic is termed a developmental trajectory, and it is governed by the interactions among risk and protective factors. This ongoing interaction means that children who start with similar characteristics may develop diverse outcomes over time (termed "multifinality"). For example, children who suffer physical abuse can have a variety of mental health outcomes as adults, and some will abuse their own children while others will not. Conversely, sometimes children start with very different characteristics but have a common outcome (termed "equifinality"). For example, depressed adolescents may have no previous psychiatric history or family history of depression, a family history of depression only, a previous psychiatric history only (e.g., an anxiety disorder or ADHD), or a psychiatric history as well as a family history of depression. Depression in a previously high-functioning teen may have a very different course and prognosis than depression that occurs in a teen who has been suffering for years with other mental health issues. The latter may require more intensive treatment to address the teen's multiple mental health issues and their adverse effects on his or her development. Finally, the same disorder may manifest differently over time (termed "heterotypic continuity"). Thus, a child with ADHD may appear very distractible in school, while an adult who has a profession that does not require much sustained attention (e.g., a salesperson) may not seem any different from her peers. Yet, other situations affected by inattention may result in functional problems in other areas, such as having a poor driving record or unpaid bills that hurt her credit rating. It is also important to note that children's development does not necessarily proceed at the same rate for different aspects of their growth. For example, if there are two children of similar age, one may be advanced academically but socially immature, while the other may struggle with academics but behave more maturely with peers.

Understanding these variations in development is critical when working with children and providing guidance to their parents. For example, in treating the two children previously mentioned for anxiety, the therapist might want to role-play social situations with the child who is socially immature and spend more time assisting with the cognitive aspects of treatment in the child with academic difficulty. Parents would need to be cautioned differently about the limitations of treatment in each case and given different advice on how to support the child's progress. Interestingly, academic and social difficulty could each adversely affect self-esteem in these children (an example of equifinality).

BASIC DEVELOPMENTAL CONCEPTS RELATING TO CASE FORMULATION

For some readers, the ideas described above may raise the question "Does one have to be an expert in all aspects of normal and abnormal child development in order to do a good case formulation?" Fortunately, the answer is no. Although trying to learn more about child development is a laudable goal, knowledge in the field is expanding so rapidly that even so-called experts may not be aware of some recent findings. On the other hand, a basic understanding of how children think and what they need emotionally at various developmental stages can be very helpful in case formulation. Some of these ideas relate to theories of psychological development, which are described in detail in Chapter 4.

A few relevant developmental ideas, however, are not linked to specific theories but are instead subscribed to by most authors in the field of children's mental health (Cicchetti, 1990; Weisz & Kazdin, 2010). These include the following:

- Children are highly dependent on their environment, especially when very young.
- Families constitute children's main social influence, especially when very young.
- Aspects of children's environments outside the family (e.g., school, peer group) become increasingly important to them as they mature.
- In preadolescents, parents often define the problem that is presented to the clinician, and parents need to "buy into" (i.e., agree with and accept) the formulation and treatment recommendations if these are to be followed.
- The ability of youth to define their own problems and the need for youth to "buy into" the formulation and treatment recommendations increase as they become adolescents.
- Parents often benefit from information about what is developmentally normative for their child, and children benefit from this information as soon as they are old enough to understand it.
- Developmental norms for behavior often differ by culture and should be explored to ensure an accurate formulation and improve family engagement in treatment.
- Anticipating children's future developmental challenges can be a valuable addition to the case formulation.

Each of these ideas will now be illustrated in more detail.

Young Children and Their Environment

To understand young children's dependence upon their environment, imagine yourself as an infant. You cannot walk, crawl, or even roll over yet, so you are entirely dependent on others to provide you with food, ensure you are comfortable, and keep you safe. You can't seek out your favorite activities or experiences. Instead, experiences are brought to you. Faces lean over you, enormous hands encircle your body to lift you, clothes are pulled on and off your body, and mobiles or other moving or noise-making objects may be put in front of you to stimulate your brain (or at least that's what the adults think). Your senses may be overwhelmed by everything that is presented to you, dulled by neglect, or kept alert and calm when the level of stimulation is just right. It will probably take a while for the adults to figure out that "just right" level, so life is not always pleasant. Hopefully, though, they will keep trying to find out what you need. As they become more predictably helpful, you are calmed, and your ability to calm yourself improves too. You get better and better at regulating your internal states, and you have energy left over to observe and explore the world around you.

This idealized description begs the question "What could go wrong with this picture?" One obvious problem might be that adults fail to attend to the infant's basic needs for food, comfort, and safety. For example, a parent who is focused on his or her own psychological challenges could be unavailable to meet these basic needs for periods of time, which may result in discomfort or sometimes even life-threatening peril for the infant. In response, the infant would focus his energies on these unmet basic needs and have little left over for observing or exploring the environment. A second problem might be a parent who provides the basic necessities but misreads the infant's cues, resulting in too much or too little environmental stimulation. In this case, the infant would not be able to trust the parent to be predictably helpful and calming, and so would have difficulty learning to soothe herself. It is also possible that the infant has an unusually high or unusually low need for stimulation, or a strong preference for certain types of stimulation (e.g., light touch vs. strong touch; aversion to certain noises; preference for certain textures), making it difficult for the parent to provide what is optimal for him. A demanding sibling or other parental responsibilities can also limit the parent's ability to tailor the infant's sensory diet until it is optimal. In this case, difficulties with self-regulation could develop in the infant, which would also limit her ability to observe or explore her environment.

Family Influences in Young Children

So far, we have talked about the basic needs of infants and the sensory input provided to them. To understand the socializing influence of families, however, we must imagine how these events influence young children's thoughts about the world and themselves. Different theorists have described such thoughts as "schemas" or "internal working models" (Bretherton & Mulholland, 1999). These terms relate to the same concept: young children's experiences with their families create templates for their thoughts about all relationships, and about the world. In other words, when children are young, their family's world is the only world they know, so they assume that it reflects reality outside as well as inside the family. For example, if (as an infant or toddler) my parents ignore me whenever I cry or seek their attention, then I approach relationships with the assumption that others are not interested in helping me and I must fend for myself. Consequently, I may not value close relationships very much and not be very interested in others' feelings. This attitude, in turn, may cause others to avoid getting close to me, confirming my assumption that others are not interested in helping me, and reinforcing my emotionally distant, self-reliant attitude in a self-perpetuating pattern. These ideas are elaborated in the section on attachment theory in Chapter 4.

Even in the presence of secure parent–child relationships, children can struggle with distorted views of themselves and others. For example, the child who is temperamentally very different from his siblings or parents may feel like he doesn't belong in the family and therefore question his place in the world. Thus, a musical prodigy may feel out of place in a very athletic family, and an exceptional athlete may feel uncomfortable in a family of musicians. Children who have been adopted or separated from their families for long periods of time sometimes share these feelings of being an outsider.

On the positive side, families can help young children modify temperamental tendencies to allow for better social adaptation. For example, children who have an inhibited temperament (aversion to new people and new situations) are predisposed to anxiety disorders, but most do not develop them. It is thought that in most cases parents patiently encourage and support their inhibited child in facing new situations, allowing the child to gradually develop the ability to deal with such situations independently. Similarly, parents who deal with tantrums or other misbehavior by calmly setting limits (e.g., using a short time out) often help the child gradually control that behavior.

Influences Outside the Family

Once children begin to attend day care or kindergarten, they are obviously exposed to social influences outside the family. As they mature, these influences grow increasingly important to children, but the confidence to deal with them successfully usually requires family encouragement and support. New environments can be a source of stress (e.g., conflict with teachers or peers, learning difficulties) or present new opportunities. For example, academic or athletic success can be a source of self-esteem for some children; exposure to a caring, encouraging teacher can help heal some of the emotional wounds left by negative family experiences.

When there is a discrepancy between family expectations and the expectations of school personnel or friends, for example, children may feel plunged into feelings of uncertainty, confusion, or distress. Many children experience such discrepancies at adolescence as they begin to experiment with behaviors that may conflict with parental norms. Most parents of teenagers have found themselves saying at least once, "If all your friends were jumping off a cliff, would you?" or making some similar frustrated comment. Adolescents often oscillate between identifying with their peer group's expectations and the expectations of their parents, and most eventually come to a resolution that they are comfortable with.

Young children, on the other hand, are typically much more distressed by discrepant expectations. This can be particularly poignant in children of parents who have recently immigrated to North America. The child may want to fit in at school and with peers and feel embarrassed by parental customs or culturally based attitudes. The parents, on the other hand, may fear losing their cultural identity in the North American "melting pot," resulting in fervent adherence to their cultural practices. Some schools do celebrate cultural diversity by, for example, having an international food day or noting religious holidays from multiple faiths on the calendar. Too often, though, children who stand out because of their religious or cultural background are still made to feel awkward and torn between their families and the "new world."

Preadolescents and Mental Health Care

When preadolescent children are brought to a mental health practitioner, they face yet another new environment, and, understandably, they are usually wary of this environment. Therefore, it is not uncommon for parents to do most of the talking during a mental health assessment of a preadolescent child. Moreover, the parent often brings the child to the practitioner with certain unspoken expectations. These expectations may or may not coincide with the practitioner's formulation and treatment expectations.

One common expectation is that, similar to a family doctor, the mental health practitioner will diagnose a problem within the child, and the solution to the problem will be something that the mental health practitioner does to or with the child. Even though they rarely say so, these parents are thinking, "Here's my child, Doc. Go ahead and fix her." Meanwhile, the mental health practitioner is thinking, "The factors contributing to this problem relate to the child, the child's environment (including the family environment), and the relationship between them." Thus, treatment recommendations can be focused on the child, the parent, the relationship between the child and the parent, on other family relationships, or on school or other environments outside the family. Moreover, even those recommendations that focus on the child may require considerable parental support or encouragement. Thus, one or both parents are almost always actively involved in the treatment, and the practitioner can "fix" very few problems without them.

It is important to be explicit about these issues and ensure that children and parents understand their respective roles in treatment. Sometimes, providing facts about how the treatment works is helpful. For example, CBT requires "coaching" of new skills both within the office (by the therapist) and outside the office (by the parents), and lots of practice (by the child). Similarly, most medications require regular parental reminders if they are to be taken consistently and parental observation of their children to determine medication benefits and side effects. Behavior management requires that parents refrain from becoming angry or upset because such emotional reactions provide attention to the child and thus inadvertently reinforce bad behavior.

Sometimes, treatment discussions are not limited to facts. This may occur either when parents have strong opinions about the treatment their children need or when they need treatment for their own mental health problems in order for their children to improve. For example, in the case described at the beginning of this chapter, Malcolm's mother was strongly opposed to using medication to treat his ADHD. Considerable discussion would have been needed to explore the reasons for this opinion, their validity, and any room for negotiation. Parents may be upset by the suggestion that they themselves require treatment since they expect the therapy to focus on the child. However, when gently reframed as a means of helping their child, the suggestion sometimes becomes more acceptable. However, considerable diplomacy and more than one discussion may be needed. Some parents recognize the need for personal mental health care after struggling (often with limited success) to support their child's treatment.

Adolescents and Mental Health Care

When adolescents present with mental health problems, most practitioners report that they are more difficult to engage in treatment than younger children. Perhaps it is more accurate to say, however, that they disengage from treatment more easily than younger children. Adolescents are often adults in physical, if not emotional, stature and more autonomous than younger children, so it is usually not possible for parents to force them to attend treatment sessions, and some adolescents will deliberately avoid treatment in order to defy parental wishes or assert their autonomy. Even if distressed by symptoms, adolescents may deny their problems or be reluctant to seek treatment because of a fear of the stigma that may be associated with mental health treatment in their peer group. Some adolescents will recognize their problems and be motivated to work on them, but these are in the minority.

To engage adolescents, practitioners often need to phrase various aspects of the formulation in terms that are relevant to them. For example, a practitioner may think that there are negative, self-perpetuating circular interactions between parent and teenager but say, "I think that when your mom nags you about homework, that bugs you so you put off doing it. [Teenager nods in agreement.] Unfortunately, the more you put it off, the more worried she gets about your grades, and the more she nags. Then, you put off doing it even more. Do you see how that might get the two of you stuck?" This explanation is not only provided in teen-friendly language but also leads nicely into a discussion of how mother and adolescent might begin to get "unstuck," and how treatment might help (e.g., family therapy).

Similarly, the treatment plan should be phrased in terms of its contribution to the adolescent's goals, not just parental goals for the adolescent. For example, parents may want treatment to improve the adolescent's behavior at home and boost school performance. The adolescent, on the other hand, may place greater value on feeling better and enjoying more activities with friends. The practitioner should not, however, presume to know the adolescent's or parents' goals. For example, some adolescents value school performance more than their parents do, and some parents value the adolescent's feelings more than good behavior. Treatment goals need to be elicited separately from parents and teenagers, and hopefully some overlap can be found. When it cannot, practitioners usually do best focusing on the adolescent's goals, as it is ultimately the adolescent who determines whether or not treatment occurs.

Education about Developmental Norms

Parents or children seen in mental health practice can have unrealistic expectations about what is considered developmentally normal or average at certain ages. When the child's development is not far from the average, informing the child and parents about this fact can be reassuring. Thus, if the child is old enough to understand, it is often helpful to say, "Many kids struggle with this at your age" or "Not everyone can do that at your age." Even when the child's development appears delayed in one area, this delay may not be disastrous depending on its importance. For example, parents sometimes assume that because their friends' children all started going to summer camp after third grade, their child should be able to do the same. If the child is unable to do so, this is inconvenient to the parents (as they must find an alternative plan for the summer) but may not be a cause for concern if there are no other symptoms of anxiety or other emotional difficulty in the child. Furthermore, there is a wide range of "normal" for some developmental changes. For example, the "normal" age for learning to ride a bicycle can range from 4 to 8 or older. The age of onset of puberty can vary even more widely.

Sometimes, there is a therapeutic value to correcting unrealistic developmental expectations. This is particularly true when parents' expectations are clearly too high or too low. For example, parents who expect their 6-year-old to do a chore every day in order to earn a treat on the weekend are harboring unrealistic expectations. These parents may become angry when the child does not comply, thus creating interpersonal problems that could easily be avoided if they understood they have set an overly high developmental expectation. Six-year-olds have a very short concept of time, so a treat that is 6 or 7 days away is meaningless to them. Furthermore, the ability to delay gratification (rather than just stealing the treat from the cupboard) is poorly developed in most 6-year-olds. Therefore, getting angry is not only unfair to the child, it is confusing and will likely make the child feel badly about himself. Saying to the child, "When you put your dishes away, then you can have dessert" is much more meaningful than promising a bigger treat in a week's time.

Occasionally, parents have unrealistically low expectations. This sometimes occurs when they are reluctant to set limits on misbehavior that the child could control with effort. Parents may make excuses like "boys will be boys" when children engage in minor vandalism or roughhouse to the point where someone is injured. They may also want to relate to the child as a friend and leave the limit setting to someone else (e.g., the other parent or the "mean" vice principal). Regardless of the reasons, parents benefit from hearing that the ability to control behavior does not develop automatically in children. Children need consistent limits that control their behavior if they are to develop the ability to control behavior themselves in the long run. Furthermore, misbehavior is unlikely to be "outgrown" without parental intervention. Rather, small boys and girls who misbehave become big boys and girls who misbehave, and the latter are much more difficult for parents to manage.

Developmental Norms and Culture

When should children be expected to dress themselves? When should they sleep in their own beds? When should they be allowed to plan their own weekend activities and merely "check in" with parents periodically? When should they be allowed to have their own cell phones? When should they be allowed to date? The answers to these questions vary widely across and even within cultures. For example, in some cultures the answer to the last question is "never"; in others it may be "around 16, but with accompaniment." In still others there are fewer restrictions. People within the same culture may be more or less traditional, depending on the extent to which they have embraced mainstream North American culture (so-called "acculturation") and the extent to which they have retained their traditional practices and values. Also, the degree of acculturation is not necessarily related to the ability to speak English. Thus, a highly proficient English speaker may have very traditional expectations of his or her family, or not. The processes involved in becoming a responsible adult and becoming independent of one's family of origin also differ across cultures. Some cultures have rites of passage marking certain transitions (e.g., confirmation, first communion, bar or bat mitzvah); others encourage gradual exploration of adult roles. Expectations concerning mental health and mental health treatment also differ across cultures, which will be discussed more in Chapter 6.

For all of these reasons, the mental health practitioner is well advised to avoid making assumptions about developmental norms based on culture, and to openly discuss cultural values that relate to treatment with the child and parents. For example, one might ask, "In North America, children of this age would typically be doing _____. What would be expected [or allowed] in your culture?" Or, "Usually, we recommend treatment for this, but I'm not sure if you see it as a problem at this age," or "How is his or her behavior different from what you would expect or hope for at this age?" With respect to treatment, one could ask, "Usually we involve the child and the parents in this type of treatment. How would that be for you?" or "How would you hope to see your child change with treatment?" Depending upon the responses, follow-up questions could then be used to clarify specific cultural differences.

Anticipating Developmental Change

Understanding children's difficulties in a developmental context often allows the therapist to anticipate future problems. In particular, children whose problems are only partially amenable to intervention may face challenges related to their ongoing difficulties, and to increasing awareness of these difficulties. For example, children on the autism spectrum can learn to regulate certain behaviors and anxieties with treatment. However, ongoing difficulty with transitions may pose a challenge as they enter middle school, where frequent class transitions are the norm. Ongoing social awkwardness may also greatly concern these youth—and their parents—when they reach adolescence, as they become increasingly aware of being different from their peers. This awareness of being "different" and other ongoing struggles with their symptoms can predispose to adolescent depression in this population. Preparing for the challenges associated with adolescence, particularly the transition to high school, can therefore be an important contribution to the mental health of youth on the autism spectrum. Youth with ongoing anxiety, ADHD, learning disabilities, and other chronic mental health conditions often also need additional support at times of transition.

WHAT ABOUT MALCOLM?

To conclude, let's take a look at how some of these ideas might have helped Malcolm, the boy described at the beginning of the chapter. Developmentally, Malcolm is a preadolescent. Thus, his parents define the problem that is presented to the clinician, and his parents need to agree with and accept the formulation and treatment recommendations if these are to be followed. Since Malcolm's parents cannot agree on the nature of the problem, the parents' views do not correspond with those of the school, and nobody has interviewed Malcolm, the clinician is put in the position of a referee who is expected to correctly define the problem. The clinical diagnoses of ADHD and generalized anxiety disorder are partially consistent with the views of Malcolm's school and those of his mother but do not address the father's view that Malcolm is "lazy." Not surprisingly (given the lack of attention to his view), Malcolm's father does not become involved in his son's mental health care. The psychiatry resident therefore presents the treatment recommendations (without a formulation) to Malcolm's mother and pursues the part of the treatment she is willing to accept: the anxiety-focused group. Treatment for the primary diagnosis, ADHD, is not pursued in deference to the mother's wishes. In short, both the problem definition and the treatment provided have been tailored to the mother's needs, which may not be in Malcolm's best interest.

From Malcolm's point of view, his family is still an important social influence, but the opinions of his school and his peer group are becoming increasingly important. His lack of success at school will soon begin to affect his self-esteem and may result in some teasing by peers, leading to a further source of distress. Each of these problems places him at risk for further anxiety and possibly depression (due to low self-esteem) as he matures. These future developmental challenges can be anticipated, so improving Malcolm's school functioning should have been prioritized in treatment.

Apart from these developmental considerations, it would have been very helpful to gather additional information during Malcolm's mental health assessment in order to construct a formulation of his difficulties. For example, the fact that Malcolm's anxiety symptoms are so consistently linked to the school day suggests a need to investigate school problems in more detail. Learning disabilities are a biologically based factor that often contributes to both inattention and anxiety symptoms. Overly critical teachers and bullies are common environmental sources of distress at school. Children from certain cultural or religious groups can experience discomfort with secular ideas and attitudes in the public school system. Any of these could contribute to Malcolm's morning stomachaches.

Parental disagreements about the nature of children's problems are often a clue to other types of family conflict. Therefore, it would have been helpful to interview Malcolm alone and ask him about how people in his family get along. The practitioner also could have made an effort to reach Malcolm's father and obtain his perspective on the family. It is even possible that most of Malcolm's symptoms relate to worry about his conflicted family or (in the case of child abuse or domestic violence) traumatic memories affecting his ability to attend at school.

The strong opposition to medication voiced by Malcolm's mother also deserves further exploration to allow for the opportunity to address her concerns. Sometimes, such opposition is based on misinformation about medication garnered from friends or the media. Sometimes, it is based on cultural or religious views that discourage or prohibit the use of psychotropic medications. Sometimes, the reasons are more personal. For example, Malcolm's mother might have had a negative experience with psychotropic medication herself. Alternatively, she might have an acrimonious relationship with Malcolm's school and feel that giving Malcolm medication for ADHD represents an acknowledgment that the school was right about her son and she was wrong. It is worth inquiring about each of these possibilities.

Finally, a good formulation would have revealed factors that might perpetuate Malcolm's problems, as well as factors that might be protective. Sadly, one of the likely perpetuating factors in this case would be the treatment itself. Malcolm's inability to succeed in the anxiety-focused group treatment mirrors his inability to succeed at school and would probably increase his anxiety and further decrease his self-esteem. Protective factors might include personal strengths or supports that are not obvious from the diagnostic interview. For example, Malcolm might have the ability to make friends, an athletic or musical ability, or a supportive relationship with an encouraging teacher or coach.

It may seem like a great deal of extra time would be needed to elicit all of this extra information, but this is not always true. As we will see in the next chapter, an astute clinician can use interviews, questionnaires, and other investigations selectively to ensure a thorough understanding of the child's difficulties in a reasonable period of time.

CHAPTER 2

Gathering Relevant Information

Key Assessment Strategies

To understand the importance of gathering key information before attempting to formulate a case, think of the process of formulation as being similar to solving a clue in a crossword puzzle. Let's say it is a five-letter word, the clue is "precedes a fall," and you know the fourth letter is "d." Given this somewhat obscure clue and only one letter, you might struggle. Then you discover the second letter is "r." Is it still difficult? There's a silent "e" at the end. Does that make it clearer? The first letter is "p." Most people, at this point, would recognize the word "pride" and the biblical saying "pride goeth . . . before a fall." The final letter is relatively easy to figure out when you know the other four.

Similarly, practitioners require a number of pieces of information to successfully formulate a case. Missing one or two pieces is not necessarily disastrous, but if substantial amounts of information are missing, formulation may not be possible or the formulation may be inaccurate. Using the puzzle analogy, if you only knew the clue "precedes a fall" and the letters "d" and "e," you might guess "slide" rather than "pride."

At the same time, it is important to be efficient in gathering and organizing information to streamline the assessment and formulation process and ensure that important treatment decisions can be reached in a timely manner. Lengthy assessments that postpone treatment can prolong children's suffering and sometimes alienate families to the point where they seek help elsewhere. Therefore, this chapter highlights key assessment strategies and methods of effectively and efficiently gathering information relevant to case formulation.

SOURCES OF INFORMATION

As mentioned in the previous chapter, the information needed to formulate a case focuses on biological, psychological, social, and spiritual factors that are relevant to the child's difficulties. Some of these factors contribute to the difficulties, while others ameliorate or protect from the difficulties. The assessment process seeks information about both risk and protective factors in each area.

Such information can come from a variety of sources. These can include interviews with the child and various family members, standardized questionnaires, the therapist's reactions to the child and various family members, interviews or reports from people outside the family, such as the child's teacher(s), and additional investigations. Each of these sources will be discussed in turn. Before doing so, however, it is important to consider the assessment structure. In other words, the practitioner should think about who should participate in the assessment and what information can be elicited in a group interview versus an individual interview.

ASSESSMENT STRUCTURE

Interviewing several people at a time can reduce assessment time and provide important clues about the nature of the relationships among those people. On the other hand, people are unlikely to publicly disclose sensitive types of information. For example, adolescents are unlikely to reveal substance use or antisocial activities in front of their parents. Children who have been abused by a parent are unlikely to disclose this information in the presence of the perpetrator. Similarly, parents may be reluctant to discuss their personal or family psychiatric history in front of their children. Family secrets (e.g., an impending separation or divorce, the serious illness of a family member, or a family member going to prison) are also often not shared with young children, and yet these outlying factors may influence their mental health profoundly. For this reason, the open-ended question "Is there anything happening in your family that you didn't want to discuss in front of your child/ parents?" is critical to include in every child and parent interview. In addition, people are often reluctant to express discrepant opinions in a group, and perceptions of children's difficulties are known to vary widely by informant (reviewed in Barbosa et al., 2002). Thus, children may experience more or fewer symptoms than their parents describe, or one parent may have a completely different view of the child's difficulties than the other. These differences are less likely to be elicited in family interviews than individual ones.

Ideally, the practitioner would interview all family members individually and as a group, but this process may result in an unnecessarily lengthy assessment. Therefore, it is common practice to interview the child who is presenting with difficulties, the child's parents, and the parents and child together. This represents a reasonable compromise, though it does miss potentially valuable information from siblings and information one parent may not wish to disclose in the presence of the other parent. An astute clinician will follow up with additional interviews in these areas if indicated, for example, by obvious discomfort on the part of one parent when talking in the presence of the other. Additional interviews may also be indicated if there are people living in the same household (e.g., grandparents or other members of the extended family) who have daily contact with the child and parents and can add potentially valuable information.

When obtaining assessment information from parents, it is often easier to arrange interviews with one parent (typically the mother) than with both parents together. In single-parent households, this is obviously necessary. However, if two parents are involved in raising the child, then it is prudent to interview them both. Although this practice may be inconvenient for parents, it clearly sends the message that both parents' views are important and that both have an important role to play in their child's care. Interviewing both parents improves the chances of obtaining unbiased information and can also improve parental participation in any treatment proposed. If one parent has not had the opportunity to express his or her views, that person may have limited motivation to participate. The likelihood that both parents will agree to and become appropriately involved in a treatment plan is higher if both have been involved in the assessment process from the start.

If both parents cannot be seen at a particular time, it is worthwhile to arrange a separate interview for the nonattending parent. Providing babysitting for siblings so that both parents are free to participate in the assessment or offering to discuss the child's difficulties by telephone with the nonattending parent are other potentially helpful options.

Separate interviews with each parent are also helpful in situations where parents are involved in an acrimonious separation or divorce and therefore have difficulty remaining cordial in each other's presence.

Given the time required for a thorough assessment, clinicians sometimes question the value of interviewing the family (or at least the parents and the child presenting with difficulties) together. If the only purpose of a child mental health assessment were to question each informant, then the value of a family interview would be limited. However, observing family interactions usually yields a large amount of additional information, as described in the "Information from the Interview Process" section below. Put simply, there are often differences between what people say in response to questions and what they do. For example, a parent may say, "My child has terrible separation anxiety, even though I really try to reassure her." During the family interview, however, the child sits in the parent's lap and is returned to the parent's lap whenever she tries to climb down. This behavior suggests that there is anxiety about separation in the parent as well as the child.

Interviewing the family together also affords the clinician the opportunity to adapt to family expectations. For example, in some cultures it is considered rude to address children before addressing parents. When the family is interviewed together, the clinician can ask, "I understand we're here to talk about problem X. Who would like to tell me about that?" or "Who would like to start?" This approach is respectful of the family's traditions and also provides useful information about family dynamics, as the family spokesperson is usually in a position of some power. Also, young children are often more comfortable beginning the assessment process in the presence of their parents.

INFORMATION FROM THE INTERVIEW CONTENT

When conducting interviews in child mental health assessment, clinicians typically multitask: they ask questions relevant to the child's difficulties (the interview content), and they observe the child and parents' behaviors as they are being interviewed (the interview process). Both are important sources of information, but let's start with a discussion of interview content.

To begin, the clinician is more likely to elicit relevant content if she takes the time to put the child and family at ease and make a connection with both the child and the parents (often called "establishing rapport"). Some requirements are obvious: presenting yourself as warm, relaxed, and open, cordially inviting people into the office, ensuring that everyone has a comfortable place to sit, making sure that the room is at a comfortable temperature, nobody is hungry or needs to visit the bathroom, the door is closed for privacy, and the interview is free from interruptions. Any obvious discomfort should be addressed before starting, or whenever it is noticed. For example, a parent who checks his watch may be worried about a parking meter about to expire or about not missing too much work. Gently comment on the behavior and address the concern (e.g., "I see you're looking at your watch. Do you have a time constraint?"). Ask that any electronic devices (e.g., cell phones, pagers, handheld video games) be turned off or placed in silent mode.

Sitting around a table often seems more relaxed than peering across a desk at your clients. Providing a structure for the assessment also helps put people at ease. For example, a clinician can say, "I usually like to talk about the issues with everyone present first to get a good history. Then, I will talk to [child's name] separately, and you, Mr. and Mrs. [name], separately because parents and children sometimes see things differently. At the end, we will take some time to do a summary and talk about what to do next." Mirroring the tempo and body language of the interviewees throughout the interview also helps convey that you are empathic to their concerns. If questionnaires will be part of the assessment, it is helpful to indicate when there will be time to complete these so it is clear that they should be set aside for the time being. Usually, parents have time to complete questionnaires during the child interview and children have time during the parent interview.

If a structured diagnostic interview is used, it is important to prepare families for this approach. For example, the clinician can say, "I will ask you a series of specific questions about different mental health issues. There will also be time to discuss your concerns about [child's name] more generally, but for now please answer only the questions asked." Without such preparation, the process can seem rather cold or unempathic. If a nonstructured interview is used, the clinician generally starts with open-ended questions about each person's concerns and then moves on to more specific questions based on their responses. It is important, however, to make sure that everyone is involved in the discussion at some point. While it can be tempting to focus on the most vocal participants, this practice can leave others feeling left out. Make sure to engage each quiet family member at least once in the course of the interview.

The content of the interview includes but is not limited to diagnostic information about the child's mental health symptoms. As illustrated in the example of Malcolm in Chapter 1, relying on diagnostic information alone is inadvisable. This raises the question: how does one cover the nondiagnostic aspects of the interview systematically? The biopsychosocial–spiritual model provides some guidance. One wants to explore each of the four aspects of the model, its relationship to the child's difficulties, and its evolution over the child's lifetime. The result is a list of risk and protective factors in each area from the remote past, the recent past, and from the child's current experience. The process of putting these factors together is illustrated at the end of this chapter, but for now it is helpful to use them as a guide to the nondiagnostic aspects of the interview. For example, my interest in the relationship between biology and the child's difficulties would lead me to ask about his past general health, any current or prior medical problems, and any developmental delays (remote risk and protective factors); recent illnesses, lifestyle habits, and use of prescription or nonprescription drugs (recent risk and protective factors); and current lifestyle habits as well as parental attitudes that might support good medical care and a healthy lifestyle (current risk and protective factors). Similar inquiries about remote, recent, and current factors can be made about psychological, social, and spiritual aspects of the child's development.

Because children's perceptions may differ from those of their parents, it is also important to obtain information about the nature of the problem and about family interactions separately from children and parents. Some children do not think they have problems, as parents typically initiate children's mental health assessments. Other children are as distressed or more distressed than their parents about mental health symptoms. The clinician should elicit children's descriptions of how supportive or unsupportive they find their families. If there are family conflicts or other problems in the home, children are often more willing to reveal these than their parents are. Sensitive or potentially dangerous issues should also be explored separately with children and parents. For example, children are more likely to disclose bullying by peers, violence in the home, and serious thoughts of suicide in private than in their parents' presence. Parents, on the other hand, are more likely to disclose family financial problems or potentially embarrassing family information when their children are not present.

It is also important to recognize that children's behaviors are often quite different depending on the child's environment. Thus, a child could be quite well mannered at school but difficult to manage at home. Conversely, some children exhibit abilities in the home environment, where they feel safe, that they do not exhibit at school, where they may be more inhibited. Therefore, it is important to obtain information about the child's functioning at home, at school, and with peers.

One useful approach to gathering environment-specific information is asking children and parents, "Will you take me through a typical day step by step, as if we had a video camera filming you?" With school-age children, ask about weekdays and weekends separately. Make sure that you elicit a description of what the child does, how other people around the child respond, and what the child does next. By obtaining these details, you will quickly discover helpful and unhelpful interactions between the child and his or her environments. You may need to interview the parents about details in the home environment and the teacher about details in the school environment.

For example, Stacey is an oppositional, temperamentally difficult 9-year-old girl in a single-parent household. She starts the day refusing to get out of bed, resulting in nagging by her mother, who finally yanks off her blanket to get her to move. Once up, Stacey picks at her breakfast slowly, despite her mother's efforts to make her eat more quickly. She then returns to her room to dress but instead plays a game until her mother barges in and yells at her to get a move on. By this point, there is little time for personal hygiene, so Stacey's mother splashes water on her daughter's face, quickly brushes her teeth, and runs a brush through her tangled hair, which causes her daughter to accuse her of being "abusive." The school bus is about to arrive, so gym clothes, books, and a sandwich (prepared the night before in anticipation of the morning rush) are thrown together in a bag that Stacey drops on the stairs on the way out. Fortunately, the bus driver waits for her, and Stacey's mother breathes a sigh of relief as she departs.

After school, Stacey drops her coat and bag on the floor, grabs a cup of pudding, and plops herself in front of the television for half an hour to unwind (as there is "hell to pay" if she is not allowed this time, according to her mother). Despite this downtime, Stacey and her mom start arguing about her homework, which needs to be done before Stacey goes to her swimming lesson. Homework is eventually begun but not finished before the lesson, so there is more heated discussion about homework after she returns home. At dinner Stacey eats well but teases her younger brother, who complains to his mother. Stacey's mother admonishes her to stop, but she continues to tease. Bedtime is "a nightmare," according to the mother, as Stacey drags out the bedtime routine even more than the morning routine. On Saturday, Stacey's mother is exhausted, so she lets her watch television and sleep "whenever" so she can catch up on her housework and attend to her son. On Sunday, Stacey's mother drags her daughter to church (after another difficult morning routine) and engages in more "homework battles" with her. "Then on Monday things start over again, worse than ever," the mother concludes.

This very unpleasant scenario illustrates a very common and very ineffectual parent–child interaction pattern: the nagging parent and the irresponsible child, who habitually interact in a negative way. The lack of effective discipline and the lack of any positive parent–child interactions must both be addressed if this situation is to improve. Stacey's teasing of her brother may relate to her envy of the brother's more positive relationship with the mother, rather than representing a separate problem. Irregular sleep cycles also merit attention, as they are probably exacerbating the situation for both mother and daughter. It would be interesting to obtain a similar "step by step" description from Stacey's teacher to determine if her behavior is better at school, suggesting that it is amenable to changes in the environment, and also to elicit strengths she may exhibit in the school environment. Thus, asking about the "typical day" not only provides a rich, detailed description of problems but can also provide important clues about where and with whom intervention is most likely to be fruitful.

INFORMATION FROM THE INTERVIEW PROCESS

When interviewing children and parents, you often learn as much or more from what they do than from what they say. Therefore, stepping back and observing the interview process can yield critical information for any child mental health assessment. Such observations can focus on the behaviors of each individual being interviewed, interactions among pairs of individuals being interviewed (e.g., parent–child interactions or interactions between the child's parents), and family interactions.

Most clinicians are already making observations about the individual child as they evaluate his or her mental status (reviewed in Tomb, 2008). When observing the child, one can note abnormal movements (e.g., tics); unusual mannerisms (e.g., stereotypies that commonly occur in autism); tense or relaxed facial expression and body posture; and restlessness (common in ADHD) or very slow movements (common in depression). The rate, prosody, and clarity of speech are also informative. For example, mood disorders can slow or accelerate the rate of speech, tone of voice may be unusual in children on the autism spectrum, and stuttering or articulation problems may result in embarrassment or teasing of the child, affecting self-esteem. The child's vocabulary can give clues to his or her level of cognitive development but can also reflect shyness, struggling with a new language, or (in the case of stilted or precocious vocabulary) a lack of awareness of social norms (e.g., in children with high-functioning autism). The child's responses to open-ended questions can vary from silence (in children who are defensive or overly self-conscious) to very detailed, circumstantial descriptions (in children who are either unfocused or anxious about failing to include enough information). Losing track of the question entirely or talking about unrelated matters is a very concerning sign, as this may indicate a thought disorder associated with psychosis. Some defiant children, however, can also provide unusual answers or deliberately avoid answering questions altogether. Children can also be distracted during the interview by noises or objects in the office (common in ADHD) or by internal stimuli (common in psychotic states and in some autistic children). No one observation is diagnostic, but taken together they provide clues to the nature of the child's difficulties.

The emotions expressed or not expressed during an interview are often very informative. For example, a child may claim that something is not upsetting but avert his gaze or shift uncomfortably in his chair when asked about the issue. In this case, the clinician should trust the child's body language more than the child's words. Sudden tears in response to a question always warrant a discussion (after providing some tissues, of course). Gently acknowledge the upset feelings and ask what went through the child's mind that prompted the emotions. If the child can't say, hazard a guess. An accurate guess is usually experienced as very empathic, and an inaccurate one can be somewhat empathic if you follow it by saying, "It must be hard when people can't understand what you're going through." At this point, though, the practitioner should usually move on to another topic, as the purpose of assessment is to gather information, not to delve into painful emotional issues that cannot be fully addressed before the child leaves your office.

Noting the predominant emotion and the range of emotional

expression is also important. Most mentally healthy children are nervous on entering the clinician's office but have a predominantly positive mood after a few minutes as they feel more at ease. Persistent anxious, angry, or negative mood during the interview suggests emotional
problems might be present in these areas. Elated or rapidly changing
emotions can occur in mania or in children abusing certain street drugs.
A narrow range of emotional expression is common in depression and
also in some forms of psychosis. Emotions clinicians observe can thus
provide valuable clues to the child's psychological problems, though
none are diagnostic. Finally, we must recognize that children's emotional reactions to clinicians may mirror their reactions to important
adults in their lives (i.e., their parents). For example, children raised
by critical parents may try to please the clinician or take a long time to
respond due to fear of the clinician's reaction. By contrast, children who
are in conflicted relationships with their parents may behave defiantly,
seeing the clinician as the parents' ally.

Each of these observations can be made in the parent as well as
in the child interview. In addition, parents often come with implicit
hopes or expectations regarding the outcome of the assessment. It is
important to make these explicit by asking, for example, "What do you
hope will happen by the end of today's meeting?" or "Do you have an
opinion regarding what would be most helpful for your child?" The
answers can vary widely and often reveal culturally based expectations of mental health care and readiness to engage in various forms
of treatment. For example, in some cultures parents expect the practitioner to tell them what to do and send them on their way, rather than
forming an ongoing therapeutic relationship, whereas in other cultures
parents feel they have not been taken seriously unless the practitioner
suggests ongoing therapy. Some parents bring their child for a mental
health assessment expecting a certain type of treatment and are angry
and disappointed if this treatment is not recommended. For example,
in my own practice I often see parents who insist that their child needs
CBT, even if the child is not well suited for this therapy and could
instead benefit from another form of treatment. Talking about these
issues openly early in the assessment can often avoid hurt feelings at
its conclusion.

Whenever two or more people are interviewed together, the clinician can observe the relationships among them. Some aspects of these
relationships are obvious. For example, the child who clings and cries
when separating from a parent in order to engage in an individual

interview probably suffers from separation anxiety in relation to that parent. Other aspects of interpersonal relationships are more subtle. They may include small gestures that indicate like or dislike of the other person, signs of deference to the other person (suggesting that he or she has more power in the relationship), and more or less effective communication styles. Observing these dimensions of family functioning is helpful, as they may provide clues about family members' contribution to the child's difficulties, their ability to support the child's strengths, and their ability to engage in treatment. Understanding and using these clues is discussed in more detail in Chapter 5 on social/familial factors.

For now, key observations of dyadic functioning (i.e., relationship between two people) and family functioning that can be made during the assessment are summarized in Table 2.1. These observations pertain to the degree of power various family members exert on each other, closeness and trust in the relationships, the ability to respect others' psychological boundaries and points of view, the degree of structure versus flexibility that is usual in the relationship or family, people's usual way of handling strong feelings, and the overall problem-solving style of the dyad or family. Because these ideas refer to dimensions rather than disorders, they should not be used to label relationships or families as "dysfunctional." There are many different styles of family interaction that can support children's healthy development (see Skinner, Steinhauer, & Santa Barbara, 1983). This ability to support healthy development is, from a case formulation perspective, the most important characteristic of family functioning.

The questions in Table 2.1 are designed to guide clinician observations of family functioning but are not usually asked during assessment interviews. Instead, the clinician writes relevant observations in the margins while gathering other information and organizes them after the interview ends. I often leave a wide margin on one side of the page to allow room to note such observations. After the family leaves, the observations can then be recorded in relation to the questions in Table 2.1. Sometimes the questions also prompt the clinician to remember additional details of family interaction. It is important to note that the answers to the questions represent hypotheses about family interactions and how they might affect the child. Observations from a single interview are rarely conclusive, as families may behave atypically when they know that they are being observed by a mental health professional. For example, difficulties may be dramatized by help-seeking families, or minimized by families who want to impress the clinician.

TABLE 2.1. Observations of Dyads and Families

Dimension	Observation
Power	• Who speaks first or prompts others to speak? • Who has the final say on decisions? • Whom do others try to please or persuade? • Is the child's (or children's) degree of power developmentally appropriate?
Closeness	• Do family members sit close together? Which ones? • Do family members defend each other's interests? Which ones? • Do family members seem to trust each other? Which ones?
Respect	• Do family members interrupt, criticize, or embarrass each other? Which ones? • Do some family members speak for each other? Which ones? • Are different points of view recognized as valid? • Can family members do things independently as well as together?
Structure	• Does the family have consistent rules or traditions? • Do family members agree on the rules and abide by them? • Are the rules overly rigid or inflexible?
Role of emotions	• Do family members talk about emotions and personal matters easily? • Are family members able to help each other at times of emotional distress?
Problem solving	• Are family members able to solve problems together? • Do family members tend to avoid solving problems? • Do family members tend to argue when trying to solve problems? • Does the family struggle with solving practical problems, emotional problems, or both?

INFORMATION FROM QUESTIONNAIRES

When discussing child mental health assessment, one of the most common questions practitioners raise is "What are the best questionnaires to use?" My usual response to this question is "It depends how you use them." To determine the best questionnaire for measuring anxiety in children, for example, one can readily search a psychology database and find articles about the properties of various relevant questionnaires such as their reliability, different aspects of validity, the appropriate age groups in which to use the questionnaires, the kinds of children used to generate the norms for them, and so on. Most of the ineffective use of questionnaires, however, is not due to using "bad questionnaires" but rather due to using questionnaires in ways that are ill informed.

To use questionnaires effectively, a few ideas may be helpful. First, a questionnaire represents someone's *opinion* about his or her own (or someone else's) symptoms. That opinion may or may not correspond to reality and may or may not correspond to others' opinions about the symptoms. In fact, the correspondence between questionnaire scores for symptoms children self-report and symptoms their parents report about them is usually fair to poor (Barbosa et al., 2002). Reasons for this include: children's or parents' difficulty reading or comprehending the questions (something an astute clinician will assist with if needed); children's minimization or exaggeration of their symptoms (because of defensiveness, oppositionality, anxiety, or a desire to avoid or obtain help); parents' minimization or exaggeration of their children's symptoms (for similar reasons); parents' difficulty evaluating certain symptoms because they pertain to the child's inner world; and children's difficulty evaluating certain symptoms because they pertain to others' perceptions of their behavior.

Second, *severity* on a questionnaire is measured relative to hundreds of people who have completed that questionnaire and does not necessarily correspond to severity of functional impairment or diagnosis. For example, a child may score in the "clinical" range on an anxiety questionnaire but not meet criteria for an anxiety disorder because her day-to-day activities are not hampered by anxiety. Conversely, a child may score in the "normal" range on the same questionnaire because of a desire to minimize symptoms and perhaps avoid treatment but meet criteria for an anxiety disorder because of avoidance of her daily activities.

Third, in order to avoid creating unduly long questionnaires, the *range of symptoms* that a given questionnaire measures is always a compromise between breadth and depth. Some questionnaires (e.g., broad screening measures) cover a wide range of symptoms but do not ask for many details of each type of symptom. Others (e.g., measures specific to one disorder) focus on a narrow range of symptoms in great depth. Each can be useful in different situations, as indicated below.

These ideas beg the question "How can one use questionnaires effectively in assessing children?" What follow are some common uses and practical suggestions:

- Use standardized questionnaires only in the age group for which they were designed and assist with reading and comprehension if needed. Also, the child with a developmental delay or severe learning disabilities may not be able to provide valid responses until somewhat older than the lower end of the age range for a given questionnaire.

- Use a broad questionnaire (e.g., the Child Behavior Checklist [Achenbach, 2012]) when screening for difficulties that may or may not be present; use a focused, disorder-specific questionnaire when a diagnosis is suspected based on interviews (e.g., the Children's Depression Inventory 2 [Kovacs, 2004] when suspecting depression, or the Multidimensional Anxiety Scale for Children [March, 2004] when suspecting an anxiety disorder).

- Some symptoms occur more in one environment than in another, so include informants from every environment where symptoms occur. For example, teacher reports (e.g., the Conners 3rd Edition [Conners, 2008]) as well as parent reports are needed when suspecting ADHD.

- Avoid overburdening children and parents with questionnaires (fatigue can reduce the validity of responses) by not administering questionnaires merely because you consider it "routine practice"; have a reason for administering each measure.

- Use questionnaires to supplement interview information, not to replace it, and never base a diagnosis solely on a questionnaire.

- Some children acknowledge more symptoms verbally and others acknowledge more on questionnaires, so use both and gently ask the child if he or she can talk about any new symptoms revealed on questionnaires.

- Repeat questionnaires that are specific to the child's diagnosis at intervals to monitor change. For example, a score on a standardized depression questionnaire at assessment can be considered a "baseline" measure of depressive symptoms, which may change every few weeks as treatment becomes effective. Sometimes children and parents forget how bad the initial symptoms were and assume treatment is unhelpful until they can see that small improvements are already detectable on questionnaire.

- Use discrepancies between parent and child questionnaire reports to inform practice. For example, a high level of symptoms by child report relative to parent report can indicate a highly distressed child, a lack of parental empathy for the child's distress, or both. A low level of symptoms by child report relative to parent report can indicate a defensive or oppositional child, an overly anxious parent, or both. Elevated symptom reports often (though not always) correspond to a desire to obtain treatment for those symptoms. Conversely, low symptom reports in both child and parent sometimes occur when children are referred for assessment by schools or child protective services and neither child nor parent is really interested in treatment.

INFORMATION FROM YOUR OWN REACTIONS

A potentially valuable source of assessment information that is often overlooked is your own reactions to the child, parents, or family. Sometimes these are prompted by the practitioner's personal background and biases. For example, I often find myself becoming irritated with people who portray themselves or their children as helpless victims and blame people outside the family for all of the child and family's difficulties. In part, this is due to my clinical observation that children in such families rarely make progress, and eventually the practitioner is blamed for the child remaining stuck; however, it may also relate to events in the distant past in which people close to me "played the victim" at my expense. It is important to be aware of our personal biases (with the aid of personal psychotherapy if needed) so that we can avoid unfair negative reactions to our clients and their families.

Regardless of one's personal biases, however, some children and parents consistently elicit particular reactions from those around them. Therefore, before concluding an assessment it is often worth asking oneself, "How would I react if I were the teacher, parent, or peer of this child?" and "How would I react if I had to live with this person as my parent or my spouse?" and "How would I react if I were a teacher dealing with this parent?" The answers can be very helpful in understanding how certain problems develop and what interpersonal problems might be perpetuating them.

These answers can also help us develop empathy for children and parents who present with difficult behavior, particularly if we remember that there are usually reasons for "unreasonable behavior." For example, several years ago I was confronted by a parent who was constantly accusing me of not doing enough to help her adolescent daughter, Amelia. She seemed so focused on blaming me for the lack of progress that she set very few rules and age-appropriate expectations for Amelia. Perhaps she was also unable to set limits for her daughter and hoped I would do so. Predictably, the teen's behavior deteriorated. Amelia skipped school, stayed out past curfew, experimented with various drugs, and was eventually arrested for shoplifting. The mother's conclusion after the arrest was, once again, that I had done too little to help her daughter. Exasperated, I labeled her (in private) with various unflattering personality disorders, commented to colleagues involved in the case about how "enmeshed" the family dynamics were, and generally tried to distance myself from the family, which only resulted in more (now legitimate) accusations of doing too little to help the girl. Other practitioners who had encountered this family before generally agreed with my impressions, suggesting that my reaction was not idiosyncratic.

For some reason, this mother repeatedly sought help for her child but then alienated the people who tried to be helpful. The reason became evident when digging through the first of four volumes that comprised Amelia's chart: Amelia was born shortly after her brother tragically died in infancy. The mother had brought the brother to the emergency department, had been falsely reassured and sent home, and the boy had died that night. With a newborn (Amelia) to look after a few days later, the mother had never had a chance to grieve. Instead, she became highly protective of her new daughter and highly suspicious of all health care providers, a pattern that had persisted to the present. Fourteen years later, I was (unfortunately) unable to change the pattern, but I did regard this family with less animosity and greater patience than before.

FURTHER INVESTIGATIONS

Further investigations, beyond the interviews and questionnaires I have discussed, are indicated when symptoms occur in environments outside the home (most commonly school), when one suspects difficulty in an area that cannot be assessed fully in the office, or when the severity or course of illness doesn't seem to make sense based on the available information. As previously mentioned, teacher reports can be very valuable in assessing the presence or absence of ADHD. However, teachers can also be valuable informants regarding other symptoms evident in the classroom (e.g., unusual behaviors or rituals, anxiety that is specific to tests or performance situations, deterioration in previous academic abilities) and also some symptoms evident on the playground (e.g., isolation from or aggression toward peers, clinginess with the teacher on duty). One must recognize, however, that certain playground behaviors, particularly bullying, may occur outside the teachers' awareness. Teachers can also provide an alternative, sometimes less-biased perspective on the child's difficulties than parents can. For example, teachers sometimes identify capabilities in children that parents are not aware of. Alternatively, a detailed teacher report may be helpful in challenging parents who minimize their children's difficulties.

It is also often useful to investigate whether a child has had a recent physical examination by a pediatrician or family doctor. Undiagnosed physical illnesses sometimes contribute to or even cause mental health problems, an issue that is detailed further in Chapter 3. For example, children or adolescents who are anemic, have low thyroid levels, or have recently contracted infectious mononucleosis may present with symptoms of depression. These physical problems are therefore worth ruling out before treating the young person for depression. In other cases, physical problems may contribute to teasing or ostracism by peers and are therefore worth addressing. For example, problems with articulation or stuttering warrant assessment by a speech–language pathologist; problems with gross or fine motor coordination may require the aid of an occupational therapist (assuming the doctor finds that these are chronic and not part of a new neurological problem).

A sudden onset of symptoms is usually a cause for concern and further investigation. For example, a previously outgoing child who suddenly becomes withdrawn and anxious may have experienced a traumatic event, been exposed to a new medication or drug, or be suffering from a new onset of mood disorder. Unexpected changes in demeanor usually indicate a profound change either in the child's body or in his or her environment so therefore warrant thorough investigation. The new onset of psychotic symptoms always warrants detailed medical investigations.

A deterioration in the child's previous level of functioning is also a cause for concern. Sometimes, such deterioration is secondary to the child's main mental health problem, but sometimes there is a genetic or physical cause. For example, Rett syndrome is a genetic condition in which girls appear to have symptoms of autism, but their developmental level progressively deteriorates year by year. Certain metabolic diseases can also be associated with mental health symptoms and follow a deteriorating course.

Overall, any sudden or unexplained change in the child's day-to-day functioning warrants further investigation. A useful corollary is that not every symptom or change needs to be investigated in detail. By targeting investigations to those areas where the child's presentation doesn't make sense, one avoids unnecessary or overly lengthy investigations.

ORGANIZING THE INFORMATION

Organizing the information gathered into a coherent formulation is the subject matter of the remainder of this book. This chapter concludes with an example that illustrates how you can begin this process. Figure 2.1 shows a formulation grid that can be used to record and organize information by type (biological, psychological, social, and spiritual/ cultural) and by time of occurrence (remote past, recent past, current). It can be photocopied for clinical use. Moreover, each square in the grid can include both risk and protective factors. Approaches to case formulation have traditionally emphasized the former (Kuyken, Padesky & Dudley, 2009). For example, they may speak of predisposing (remote

Time	Type of Risk or Protective Factor			
	Biological	Psychological	Social	Spiritual (including cultural)
Remote past				
Recent past				
Current				

FIGURE 2.1. Formulation grid.

risk), precipitating (recent risk), and perpetuating (current risk) factors and list "protective factors" as a fourth category. It is human nature, however, to think more about those factors to which more categories are assigned, resulting in an emphasis on risk rather than protective factors in this approach. Because it is helpful to build on children's and families' strengths in treatment, I have chosen to include risk and protective factors in all parts of the grid.

It is important to note that not every problem requires you to fill every square in the grid. For example, a child who was apparently well adjusted but recently developed a fear of flying insects after being stung by a bee has a very clear precipitant for the problem. The child's genetic predisposition to anxiety and family reactions to the sting may exacerbate or ameliorate the problem, but the formulation remains quite simple. The older the child or adolescent and the more complex and persistent the problems, however, the more all aspects of the grid become relevant to an accurate formulation. In this case, the formulation becomes a detailed story of how the problems developed and how the child developed in relation to the problems. The story explains how the biological, psychological, social, and spiritual strands of risk and resilience become interwoven over time and ultimately result in the picture presenting in your office today.

The formulation is one explanation for this picture, but it is important to bear in mind that there are usually others. Sometimes new information comes to light, resulting in alternative explanations. Other times, there are multiple ways to understand the relationships among the same risk and protective factors. This is particularly common when two factors coexist and their causal relationship is unclear. That is, it is possible that the first factor caused the second one, that the second factor caused the first, that the two factors influence and reinforce each other, or that a third factor is responsible for both. Each possibility would result in a somewhat different formulation. That is why the latter chapters of this book emphasize the importance of testing and reevaluating the formulation over time.

In Figure 2.2, a sample formulation grid is provided for a boy, Paul, who is in his early teens and presents with recent depression and a 2-year history of regular cannabis use. The clinician has recorded all relevant assessment information about Paul in the appropriate grid squares as a bulleted list. Although the list of factors and problems outlined in the grid may initially seem confusing, potential relationships among these factors readily emerge and help the clinician develop reasonable hypotheses for case formulation. The process of turning a

Time	Type of Risk or Protective Factor			
	Biological	Psychological	Social	Spiritual (including cultural)
Remote past	• Genetic predisposition to ADHD	• Insecure parent–child attachment • Mistrust of authority	• Exposure to marital conflict • Inconsistent discipline • Mother sees him as "like Dad" • No reliable parental support	• Mother's culture values education and obedience • Father's family is laissez-faire
Recent past	• Impulsive and underachieving at school • Athletic and good with his hands • Popular due to quick wit	• Drawn to antisocial peers • Identity: "I am trouble," low self-esteem • Capacity for relationships (e.g., with teacher)	• Disliked by teachers • Good, mutually supportive relationship with sister	• "Drug culture" at school
Current	• Flexible, open to new activities/ lifestyle • Drug use is hindering motivation/ energy	• Trouble keeps his parents involved to a degree • Anxious about risky lifestyle • Low self-esteem	• Parental separation • Feels he belongs with neither parent • Mother willing to give him a chance	• Drug culture includes violence

FIGURE 2.2. Sample formulation grid for Paul, a teenager with depression and cannabis use.

bulleted-list grid format into a coherent story of the child's difficulties is described in detail in Chapters 7–9, with reference to key developmental issues in (respectively) preschoolers, school-age children, and adolescents. Prior to those chapters, grids and stories are presented separately to allow emphasis on different aspects of the case formulation. Try to notice, however, how the author orders the information in the grid chronologically and then links the different biological, psychological, social, and spiritual factors in the grid in order to tell the story. Key factors from the grid are *italicized* in the story below to show how the grid and the story correspond. A case formulation can be thought of as resembling a constellation: at first it seems like a disconnected bunch of points, but soon the relationships among them become clear and you see the "Big Dipper."

Here is one possible formulation of Paul's difficulties:

Paul was the first of two children born to a married couple from very *different cultural backgrounds*. Paul's mother was a physiotherapist who was raised in a strict Asian family that placed a high value on education and obedience to one's elders; his father was a traveling salesman who was raised in a fourth-generation American family with few rules and (by his own description) a "live and let live" attitude. Although they initially joked about how "opposites attract," Paul's mother soon tired of her husband's lack of ambition and unpredictable schedule, while his father felt that his wife was "too serious, and never has any fun."

Paul's birth exacerbated their *marital stress*, as his mother felt unsupported by her husband in caring for him; the loss of her (more reliable) income added financial strain. She also reported that Paul *"was hyperactive even in the womb"* and found him challenging to parent from the start. He cried intensely and was difficult to soothe, and his mother reported, "At times, I *couldn't believe he was related to me*, let alone my son." As Paul grew into an active, distractible toddler, he also began *reminding his mother of her husband*, whom she increasingly resented. She found Paul frustrating, had difficulty showing him affection, and immediately turned her attention to his sister when she was born, just before Paul turned 2.

Paul developed into an insecure preschooler, as his father's inconsistent availability and his mother's resentment left him *without a predictably trustworthy adult*. Feeling alone and jealous of his sister, he often broke the rules either by hitting her or by stealing food from the cupboard when his mother was busy with the baby. Paul often ate to comfort himself. His mother punished him by taking away toys, sending him to his room without supper, and telling him he would be sorry when his father came home. His father would sometimes react violently to stories of Paul's misbehavior, once resulting in an emergency room visit to make sure Paul's arm was not broken. At other times, Paul's father ignored his wife's pleas to set limits for the boy. *Life at home for Paul alternated between being punished and being ignored,* with few enjoyable moments. The summer he turned 5, Paul began playing tag and "war" with boys in his neighborhood. He had fun and was pleased to find that he was a *fast runner.*

Almost immediately after starting kindergarten, however, Paul's restless nature got him into trouble. He couldn't sit still for circle time, didn't want to nap during nap time, and couldn't wait his turn for activities, which his teacher considered rude. On the playground, however, he was *popular among his peers for his athleticism and sense of humor.* He often told jokes at his teacher's expense. In the early school grades, he appeared bored and disinterested in class. Although not openly defiant, he often ignored the rules and *played games with his classmates instead of doing academic work.* His *teachers labeled him* "immature" and often sent him to the principal's office. When asked about his problems by a school social worker at the time, Paul simply said, *"I am trouble."*

At home, Paul's parents fought with increasing frequency and often in front of their children. Paul's sister was frightened by the continual arguments and ran to him for comfort. Despite his envy of her, Paul was sympathetic. *The two children became closer and more supportive of each other* over time. When the house was quiet, though, Paul's mother nagged him to do homework (which he never finished due to distractibility) and criticized his lack of discipline. He began lying about having finished his homework so that he could escape the house and be with his friends. In the preteen years, he and his friends began engaging in *vandalism and other antisocial behavior.* Paul was arrested once for shoplifting but released with a warning. His father responded by beating Paul severely. His mother responded by enrolling him in a private school "to get him away from bad influences," but his behavior did not change.

Two years ago, Paul started high school. This was initially a positive change, as he began taking a woodworking class and discovered a real talent for making things with his hands. His *shop teacher encouraged and praised* Paul's work, something he had rarely experienced at home. Unfortunately, other teachers were less charitable, and Paul's "trouble" identity soon reemerged. One of his friends introduced him to marijuana, and soon Paul was associating with a *drug-taking group of peers.* His *drug habit further reduced Paul's motivation and energy for school work,* and his grades deteriorated. Paul's parents were called to school planning meetings, arranged to have his learning assessed, and tried to better supervise his homework, but with little effect.

Eventually, *Paul's parents separated*. Paul's mother had primary custody of the children and, with her husband out of the picture, focused even more of her energies on criticizing and trying to change her son. Tired of her nagging, Paul moved in with his dad, who was often on the road for work. Unsupervised, Paul invited his drug-taking friends to the house. Unfortunately, one of Paul's friends started selling drugs out of the house, resulting in Paul having contact with even more antisocial peers and adults. One day, Paul tried to stop a fight during a *drug deal and was stabbed* in the shoulder.

While Paul recuperated in the hospital, a psychiatric consultation was obtained. Paul was diagnosed with depression, ADHD, and substance abuse. He was clearly *anxious about his risky lifestyle*, but saw *little alternative*. He concluded, "I'm no good at school, my dad is never around, and my mom hates me." He was willing to try treatment but was pessimistic about whether it would work and added, "Besides, where would I live?" *Neither parent was eager to take him back.*

The psychiatrist met with Paul and his family, and reviewed Paul's difficulties and treatment options. Not all aspects of the formulation were shared, as the family was still reeling from the shock of Paul's stabbing. However, contributing factors were discussed in general terms, and an agreement for further family meetings was obtained. After some negotiation, *Paul's mother agreed to allow him to live with her on the condition that he was treated* for his substance abuse. Treatment for all of Paul's diagnoses was undertaken, including psychotherapy to further explore and address the factors contributing to his presentation. *Paul was cooperative with treatment* and, building on his strengths, he was eventually able to complete an apprenticeship program to become a carpenter and pursue his love of sports in an amateur soccer league.

This example illustrates how a grid containing seemingly disjointed bits of information about a young person's development can be used as a scaffold for a story describing his psychological development. In an attempt to synthesize the information, a practitioner sometimes makes assumptions about the relationships among different bits of information which may or may not be correct. In Paul's case, a circular relationship between drug use and poor school performance is implied. That is, the less success Paul has at school, the more he is drawn to drugs and drug-taking peers; the more drugs he takes, the less successful he is at school. Alternatively, it is possible that, regardless of his drug use, a learning disability is contributing to Paul's school failure. Or his school failure may be almost entirely due to his ADHD. Assessing these possibilities would be important both to ensure an accurate formulation and to ensure the most appropriate care.

The testing of assumptions made in one's formulation is described further in the latter chapters of this book, and Paul's story will be revisited at that point. First, however, we examine in detail the biological, psychological, social, and spiritual components of formulation and apply them to children and adolescents of different ages.

CHAPTER 3

Biological Aspects
of the Formulation

In this chapter and the three that follow, we explore each aspect of the biopsychosocial–spiritual formulation in detail. This exploration is intended to help you review and organize potential risk and protective factors in each area before synthesizing the information from all four areas (the final step in case formulation) in a given case. Factors in each area are reviewed in depth, and key developmental considerations are noted. Chapters 7 to 9 focus on using this information with different age groups and Chapters 10 to 12 focus on different applications of the case formulation.

Biological aspects of the formulation often seem daunting, as the rapid rate of progress in medical science can make them seem inaccessible to many practitioners. Indeed, it is not possible to describe all potential biological aspects in a single chapter, or even in a single book! However, all practitioners can become familiar with common biological contributors to mental health or illness, understand how they may impact development, and know when to refer the child to a physician for more detailed investigations. These are the goals of the present chapter.

When reviewing biological risk and protective factors, it is often helpful to think about them in the following categories: constitutional factors that increase or decrease vulnerability to certain psychiatric problems; biological factors that produce psychological symptoms through direct effects on the brain; biological factors that produce psychological symptoms indirectly as the child and his or her environment respond to illness; and factors that lie at the boundary between biology and psychology. (Moreover, the impact of any factor on a child's development will vary depending on the child and family's attitudes and resources.) The form in Figure 3.1 can be used to summarize risk factors, protective factors, and their impact in the case of a child being evaluated. Later in this chapter, an example of a young girl with seizures illustrates how the figure can be completed when there are several types of biological factors at play.

There is some overlap among the factor categories. For example, diabetes can affect children's emotions owing to fluctuating blood sugar levels that impact the brain (a direct effect) and also because of parent–child conflict about appropriate management of the disease (an indirect effect). A depressed parent can be considered a constitutional

Factor Type	Risk Factors	Protective Factors	Impact on Child Development
Constitutional			
Direct effect on brain			
Indirect effects of illness			
Biological/ psychological (including somatic)			
Biological/social			
Biological/cultural or spiritual			

FIGURE 3.1. Biological factors and their impact.

risk factor for childhood depression, but negative parent–child interactions resulting from parental depression would constitute an indirect, social risk factor. Effects can also be bidirectional. For example, school failure resulting from a learning disability could predispose to substance abuse, and substance abuse can further impact learning and school performance. Conversely, school success resulting from high intelligence could protect a child from developing severe social anxiety, and being less socially anxious could contribute to further school success. Nevertheless, the categories provide a useful framework for understanding relevant biological factors, so each category will now be reviewed in turn.

CONSTITUTIONAL FACTORS

Constitutional factors are present from very early in a child's life. It is not always possible to determine their etiology: they can be due to genetic anomalies and prenatal effects, circumstances of birth, or the interaction between the child's genetic endowment and his or her earliest experiences in infancy. Clinically, parents will often report "this is the way she has always been" or "this is his personality." Developmental psychologists, on the other hand, often refer to these factors as temperament traits or aptitudes.

Protective Factors

Constitutional factors can increase or diminish the child's vulnerability to psychiatric problems, and some factors can do either depending on the child's circumstances. Those that decrease vulnerability are considered protective factors. Some common protective factors include intelligence, athleticism, musical or artistic ability, attractiveness, and a temperament that is perceived as "easy" or desirable by the parents. It is important to consistently inquire about these unique strengths and abilities. When focusing exclusively on difficulties, we compartmentalize children into diagnoses instead of understanding them as whole individuals and may miss the opportunity to build upon their strengths in treatment. For example, a boy on the autism spectrum with severe learning disabilities might have a sunny disposition and a "cute" appearance, endearing him to teachers and other adults. When providing mental health consultation to his school, one could build upon these positive attitudes toward the child in developing a plan for improving his academic progress and integration with peers.

To elicit factors that confer vulnerability, either consistently or in certain circumstances, it is important to ask about family history of psychiatric illness, the child's prenatal environment, circumstances of birth, early temperament and how the parents responded to it, and early developmental course.

Family History

The family history of psychiatric illness can reveal genetic susceptibility to certain disorders, parental worries about the child, and (in the case of psychiatric illness or other negative, abusive behavior in a parent) child exposure to less than ideal parenting practices (discussed in Chapter 5). Psychiatric genetics is a complex, burgeoning field (see Kendler & Eaves, 2005, for further details). Most psychiatric disorders are thought to be associated with multiple genes that are expressed to varying degrees. This complexity is somewhat reassuring, as a serious psychiatric illness in a family member does not necessarily doom the child to a similar fate. In fact, even in disorders with high heritability, such as schizophrenia, the risk to the child of an affected parent is 10% or less. If the affected family member is a more distant relative (e.g., a grandparent, aunt, uncle, or cousin) the risk declines considerably. Thus, parents who say "She's just like Aunt Lucille, who had to be institutionalized" can often be reassured about their child's prognosis. Nevertheless, it is important to provide accurate information, so it behooves clinicians to research the latest information on heritability when there is a potential genetic risk.

A few genetic disorders are important to recognize, as they are often linked to psychiatric or developmental problems. For the most part, these are linked to large, chromosome-based abnormalities rather than single genes. Most mental health professionals are already familiar with those involving too many or too few chromosomes (e.g., Down syndrome), and these are usually obvious enough to be diagnosed early in life. Some conditions, however, are due to abnormalities in certain parts of a particular chromosome, and these abnormalities may be more difficult to detect (Skuse & Seigal, 2008). For example, in the 22q11-deletion syndrome there is a region on chromosome 22 that is missing 20 to 30 genes. Children with this condition have a high risk of psychosis and autistic symptoms. Fragile X syndrome is an abnormality of the X chromosome that usually results in mental retardation and autistic symptoms in boys. Abnormalities of chromosome 15 can result in syndromes characterized by developmental delay and psychiatric symptoms (Angelman syndrome and Prader–Willi syndrome). An abnormality of chromosome 7, Williams syndrome, can cause intellectual impairment and unusual social behavior. Most of these syndromes, however, are associated with developmental delay and unusual facial features as well as psychiatric symptoms. Therefore, it is usually best to refer to a genetics specialist for further testing when psychiatric symptoms occur in this context.

Gene–environment interactions have received increasing attention in recent years (see Dodge & Rutter, 2011, for a helpful review). These interactions occur when a gene is considered a risk factor for a psychiatric illness only in the presence of an additional environmental risk factor. In the absence of the environmental assault, the gene does not confer a risk of psychiatric illness and may even be adaptive. Interactions that have been replicated (i.e., reported in multiple studies) to date include the link between the short allele of the serotonin-transporter-linked polymorphic region (5-HTTLPR gene) and depression in the presence of childhood maltreatment; the link between the COMT gene and antisocial behavior in the presence of ADHD; the link between the VAL variant of the COMT gene and psychosis following exposure to cannabis; and the link between the "low-activity" MAOA gene and antisocial behavior in the presence of childhood maltreatment. Although testing for these genes is not currently routine, they are likely to become increasingly important in clinical practice as researchers begin to use them to predict individual response to specific treatments (an emerging field called "personalized medicine"). There are a number of technical journals in this field, but the *Journal of the American Academy of Child and Adolescent Psychiatry* regularly reports on findings relevant to children's mental health.

Extremes of environmental deprivation or trauma, however, can impact the brain and, of course, psychological development regardless of the child's genetic endowment. Children reared in orphanages or hospitalized for long periods of time, for example, can experience failure to thrive (Spitz, 1945). Their food intake and growth is restricted in response to severe emotional deprivation. Brain development is adversely affected by malnutrition and possibly also by the faulty regulation of stress hormones that can be associated with emotional deprivation. Emotional deprivation and traumatic events early in life have been linked to alterations in stress hormone levels (Fox & Hane, 2008), placing neglected and traumatized children at risk for later psychiatric problems.

Prenatal and Perinatal History

When exploring the circumstances of the child's birth, it is helpful to begin by asking about conception and whether or not it was planned. For example, a child who is born after years of miscarriages or unsuccessful fertility treatments is likely to be highly valued by parents (and perhaps also overprotected) relative to a child who was conceived accidentally at a time when the parents were not ready to care for a baby. Prenatal care can also be compromised when pregnancy is not planned, and therefore perhaps not recognized for some time. Maternal diabetes and high blood pressure (called "preeclampsia") are common complications of pregnancy that can affect the fetus. It is also important to elicit information about maternal consumption of alcohol, cigarettes, prescription drugs, and nonprescription drugs (Hospital for Sick Children, 2012). When prenatal exposures are not known (e.g., in some adoptions or in parents who are reluctant to provide the information), it is especially important to investigate these possibilities. The effects of fetal alcohol exposure, in particular, are often missed for years, resulting in children and young adults being given unfair psychiatric labels (usually "conduct disorder") or even being jailed because the nature of their difficulties is misunderstood. There is no definitive test for this condition, but slow growth, certain facial features (small eyes, smoothing of the vertical groove above the lips, thin upper lip), and cognitive delays are common in children exposed to alcohol before birth (see *http://alcoholism.about.com/od/fas/a/fasd.htm*).

Common birth-related factors that can affect children's development include prematurity, neonatal withdrawal from any drugs the mother may have taken during pregnancy, and birth circumstances that result in lack of oxygen to the brain (Rutter et al., 2010). In severe cases the effects of these factors are obvious (e.g., cerebral palsy in the case of severe oxygen deprivation at birth). However, even if effects are not obvious at the time of assessment it is worth asking if the baby required any time in a specialized neonatal unit at birth. A history of neonatal intervention is not predictive of any particular psychiatric disorder, but rates of such intervention are increased in many disorders (i.e., it is a nonspecific risk factor). Similarly, early developmental delays and mild disabilities (e.g., developmental coordination disorder) increase the chances of children developing both cognitive and psychiatric problems later but are not specific to any particular disorder.

Temperament

Child temperament consists of patterns of behavior specific to a given child. These patterns are evident at a very early age and are therefore thought to be largely innate. Although there are many classifications of these patterns or traits, the traits originally described by Chess and Thomas (1996) included activity level, regularity, approach/ withdrawal, adaptability, intensity, mood, distractibility, persistence, and sensitivity. Children with so-called "easy" temperament typically show easy adaptation to new experiences, positive moods, and regular eating and sleeping patterns. Children with so-called "difficult" temperament typically show intense emotions, irritability, and irregular eating and sleeping patterns. Children who are slow to warm up show withdrawal from new experiences, followed by slow adaptation to them. Easy temperament is considered the most desirable by parents, as it results in the fewest stressful interactions between parent and child.

Some temperament traits are considered desirable in some families and undesirable in others. Developmental psychologists refer to this phenomenon as the "goodness of fit" between parent and child temperament. For example, a very active child might be considered less difficult to raise by active, athletic parents than by sedentary parents who prefer artistic or intellectual pursuits. Similarly, a parent who values child obedience might consider a very persistent child "willful" or "headstrong," while a parent who values the child's development of autonomy might proudly report "she has a mind of her own."

Certain temperament traits, however, do seem to place children at risk for psychiatric illness, even if there is a relatively good fit between parent and child. It is unclear if these traits represent early forms of psychiatric illness, a need for special environmental support (beyond what one would consider average parenting practices), or both. For example, children who exhibit shyness and an aversion to novelty when young (termed "behavioral inhibition") are at risk for developing anxiety disorders, particularly social anxiety disorder (Biederman et al., 2001). This temperament trait is modifiable, however, as most inhibited children do not develop disorders, and many become less inhibited over time. The tendency for most affected children to "outgrow" their inhibition is thought to relate to consistent, supportive parental encouragement to face new situations. Similarly, children who are temperamentally rigid or have difficulty regulating negative feelings may be vulnerable to behavioral problems or personality disorders over time but can improve with parenting practices tailored to their needs (Greene, 2010).

Gender

One aspect of a child's constitutional endowment that deserves additional discussion is gender. A complete discussion of gender effects on development is beyond the scope of this chapter, but several recent books provide a more detailed description (e.g., Romans & Seeman, 2006). When discussing gender effects in child development, there is often disagreement as to the extent to which these are biologically versus socially determined. For example, anxiety disorders and depression clearly increase in girls after puberty, but both hormonal and social theories have been implicated. Similarly, poor school performance in boys has been linked to both cognitive differences between boys and girls and to different social consequences of academic success for each gender. A few biological factors seem to be protective for one gender and constitute vulnerability for the other. For example, early pubertal maturation has been linked to high academic success and leadership in boys, and to low academic success in girls. Gender effects become even more complex when children are unhappy with their gender of birth (Zucker & Bradley, 1995) or struggle to come to terms with their sexual orientation.

In addition, it is important to find out if one gender or the other was desired by the parents when the child was born, as being the "undesired" gender can adversely affect the child. In some cultures, for example, there is a strong preference for male offspring. However, in some families in which there are already one or more male offspring, parents may wish for a girl. Families can also vary in how accepting they are of girls and boys who behave in ways that are consistent or inconsistent with traditional gender roles. For example, tomboyish behavior in girls and mildly effeminate behavior in boys may be severely chastised in some families and hardly noticed in others. In summary, it is important not only to consider gender as a potential risk factor for certain types of psychopathology but also to ask children about the experience of being a boy or being a girl in their particular circumstances.

DIRECT BIOLOGICAL EFFECTS

Numerous illnesses and injuries can adversely affect the brain, and therefore the child's psychological development, but several aspects of lifestyle can be protective. Regular sleep and exercise routines, for example, promote both physical and emotional health. Families often report decreases in their children's mood, anxiety, and behavior problems in response to establishing these routines.

Although the popular press has touted numerous dietary fads and dietary supplements as promoting children's mental health, the evidence in this area is far from conclusive. Emerging evidence suggests that there may be a value in limiting consumption of certain food products in certain psychiatric conditions (e.g., limiting caffeine products in anxious individuals; possibly limiting foods containing certain dyes and additives in some children with ADHD) (currently under review by the U.S. Food and Drug Administration). However, there is no clear "mentally healthy diet" that has been shown to work, so a varied diet conducive to physical health is still prudent in most cases. Dietary supplements must be evaluated in light of their potential risks and potential benefits in a given child and should not take the place of nutritious food.

Limiting children's media exposure is an increasingly important lifestyle factor in mental health. Television viewing, computer games, social media, texting, and handheld entertainment devices, among others, can add up to a great deal of "screen time" for some children. In young children, such exposure can result in direct, deleterious effects on brain development (American Academy of Pediatrics, 2012). In older children, the evidence for direct brain effects is less clear, but excessive screen time can interfere with other developmentally important activities.

Brain illnesses and injuries that can affect children's psychological development include head injuries, organic brain syndromes, and neuropsychiatric or neurodevelopmental conditions (American Psychiatric Association, 2013). Most child mental health practitioners are familiar with common neuropsychiatric or neurodevelopmental conditions, as these are treated primarily in mental health settings. In fact, as we learn more about the neurological basis of many psychiatric conditions, it is possible that we will eventually consider almost all of them to be "neuropsychiatric." Currently, however, children who have developmental delays or are on the autism spectrum are considered to have neurodevelopmental conditions, while children with ADHD,

Tourette syndrome (characterized by multiple tics), and some forms of obsessive–compulsive disorder that have been linked to streptococcal infection (called PANDAS) are considered to have neuropsychiatric conditions. Learning disabilities deserve special mention, as they often contribute to school-related psychological problems and may not be recognized for years.

Head injuries resulting in brain damage that is visible on computed tomography (CT) or magnetic resonance imaging (MRI) scans can clearly impact children's psychological development. Damage to the frontal lobes is particularly concerning, as this area of the brain helps us to sustain attention, control our impulses, and regulate our feelings. Reduced functioning in this area can therefore result in a variety of new psychological symptoms and exacerbation of preexisting ones. Mild head injuries that result in concussion (defined as head trauma with temporary loss of brain function) may not be visible on scans but can also impact cognitive and emotional development, especially if they occur repeatedly. The risk of repeated concussion in some contact sports is particularly concerning.

Neurocognitive disorders described in DSM-5 (American Psychiatric Association, 2013) can be acute (termed "delirium") or the result of a chronic illness. Delirium is a state of confusion resulting from biological processes in the brain in which the child's mental state fluctuates over the course of the day. Children can alternate between agitation and calm periods, have unusual sleep cycles, and have intermittent hallucinations or other perceptual disturbances. These symptoms only resolve when the underlying medical problem is treated.

Underlying medical problems can include diseases of the brain such as meningitis, stroke, or seizures as well as diseases affecting the whole body such as breathing or circulation problems, rheumatological diseases such as lupus, endocrine problems such as diabetes or abnormal thyroid hormone levels, and many others (Rutter et al., 2010). Intoxication or withdrawal from prescription or nonprescription drugs should be considered too. Some medications also result in frequent psychiatric or psychological side effects. For example, anti-seizure medications often impair certain aspects of thinking, bronchodilator medications for asthma can produce anxiety, and steroids can result in disturbances of mood or paranoia.

It is not important for the child mental health practitioner to know about all of these possible medical conditions, but it is useful for him or her to be aware of features that suggest a medical rather than a psychological cause for mental health symptoms. These features can be summarized in three A's: abrupt onset, associated medical symptoms, and atypical presentation of a psychological problem. For example, a child described as temperamentally "easygoing," friendly, and calm who suddenly develops intense anxiety unrelated to any apparent stress warrants investigation. Thyroid conditions can present this way, as can several other medical problems. The possibility of an undisclosed traumatic event should also be considered, however. Similarly, stomachaches that occur unpredictably and are accompanied by unexplained weight loss (a medical symptom) warrant medical investigation, whereas those that occur predictably every morning on a school day and have no associated medical symptoms do not. Unusual presentations of a psychological problem might include:

- A child who appears to regress by losing a previously established skill.
- A child who behaves "out of character" as compared to previous family and teacher observations.
- The child's symptom(s) awaken him or her from sleep.
- The child's symptoms do not vary by environment (psychological symptoms are typically better or worse at home versus at school).
- The child's symptoms are not linked to any apparent environmental trigger or change.
- There is an unusual response to psychological intervention (e.g., worsening symptoms when support is offered).

None of these features allow one to say for certain that the child's presentation has a medical basis, but they are unusual enough that a consultation with a pediatrician should be considered. In most cases, a thorough history and physical examination of the child will reveal a medical condition if one is present. Therefore, further investigations are usually targeted to conditions that are suggested by the history or physical examination. Excessive medical investigations are distressing for the child and family and can sometimes exacerbate psychological symptoms, so these should generally be avoided.

Occasionally, however, a medical problem is discovered months or even years after the original investigations are done, so it is important to maintain good communication between medical and mental health providers in these cases. In addition, one should never accuse the child of "faking" if no medical cause is found. Symptoms are distressing, whether they are due to medical causes, psychological causes, or both (see "Somatic Symptoms and Related Disorders" on pages 63–65), and we must validate that distress if we are to be helpful to the child.

INDIRECT BIOLOGICAL EFFECTS

Indirect biological effects reflect the child and family's response to the child's medical illness. These effects vary depending on the nature of the illness and its treatment, the child's previous psychological development, and the child's environment (family, school, social, cultural/spiritual). Moreover, there are sometimes bidirectional effects wherein the child and family's responses also impact the child's medical illness and its treatment. Thus, there are many possible interactions between the child, the child's environment, the illness, and medical treatment, as shown in Figure 3.2.

Subsequent chapters of this book detail children's coping styles (Chapter 4) and familial and sociocultural influences on these coping styles (Chapters 5 and 6), so only the role of medical illness and its treatment will be emphasized here. Several factors affect the psychological impact of an illness upon a child. These include the onset of the illness, chronicity, course, predictability, and its effect on life span and functionality. The latter can include physical or sensory disabilities, cognitive limitations, communication problems, difficulties with behavioral or emotional control, and social/relational disabilities (Simeonsson & Rosenthal, 2001).

One important distinction is that between the impact of congenital illness and illness that has its onset later in the course of development. The same illness or disability may affect the child in very different ways depending on when it begins. Congenital illnesses are challenging in that they often disrupt several developmental pathways. For example, children who are born blind may lag in some aspects of motor

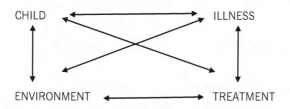

FIGURE 3.2. Indirect biological effects.

development that relate to eye–hand coordination, have difficulty reading social cues (many of which are communicated visually), and struggle with certain aspects of reasoning and problem solving that are learned primarily through sight (Chaudry & Davidson, 2001). Illnesses or disabilities acquired later in development pose different challenges. In this case, the child often struggles psychologically to adapt to life without a previously enjoyed ability, and both child and parent may experience a profound sense of loss. Simeonsson and Rosenthal (2001) provide detailed descriptions of assessment for children with different specific impairments and illnesses (motor, visual, auditory, neurological, and other special needs).

Acute illnesses are generally thought to have less psychological impact on children than those that persist for years. However, an acute illness that has long-term sequelae can be devastating. For example, children who require amputations after meningococcal meningitis must adapt to drastically different abilities after this event. Acute illnesses can also result in posttraumatic symptoms in some children, particularly if hospitalization involves a traumatic separation from a parent or other frightening events. Inquiring about details of hospital experiences is important to reveal these potential psychological scars.

The impact of chronic illness depends largely upon its course and effects on development. As mentioned, there is often a sense of grief or loss when the illness is first diagnosed. The realization that life will never again be uncomplicated by illness is difficult for many children and families. Subsequently, the predictability or unpredictability of the illness becomes an important psychological focus. Unpredictability increases anxiety in most people. Therefore, illnesses that occur unpredictably or are characterized by unpredictable crises or exacerbations can be particularly challenging. Children who suffer from anaphylactic conditions, for example, may have little day-to-day impairment, but the risk of a life-threatening reaction is a source of constant anxiety and vigilance in many of their families (Monga & Manassis, 2006). Childhood diabetes, seizure disorders, and asthma are other common medical conditions characterized by periodic crises that may not be entirely predictable or controllable. If the illness can be managed in ways that are at least partially within the child and family's control, feelings of anxiety and helplessness can often be reduced. Unfortunately, however, power struggles between parent and child can also occur around illness management.

Illnesses that predictably shorten life span or severely limit the child's long-term potential pose different challenges. Families may vacillate between anticipatory grief and desperate attempts to change an outcome that is inevitable. Further concerns arise around how much or how little to tell the child about his or her prognosis and how long to persist with various treatments, especially if these can impact quality of life, as in, for example, cognitive deterioration following cranial radiation for brain tumors (Fan, Fike, Weinstein, Liu, & Liu, 2007). Severely disabling conditions may drain family resources, prevent parents from working, and strain relationships among the nondisabled family members. Inquiring about psychosocial resources (e.g., respite care for parents) and spiritual resources (e.g., support from a religious community) is important in order to adequately support these children and families.

Treatment can also impact the child and family's development, and the child and family's participation in treatment (or lack of participation) can in turn affect the severity of the child's illness. The following story of a young girl with a seizure disorder who presented with psychiatric symptoms illustrates some of these interactions. Key points are summarized in Figure 3.3 and *italicized* in the story that follows.

Case Example: Abby

Abby was a young, initially healthy girl of average intelligence who was born into a *nurturing and protective* single-parent *family*. Her *mother had been treated for an anxiety disorder* but still described herself as "high strung." At age 10, Abby awoke from sleep one Sunday morning with a dramatic, tonic-clonic *seizure*. Her mother witnessed the seizure and called an ambulance, and Abby was taken to hospital. The attending physician initially *minimized the mother's concerns* and was about to discharge Abby, but then she had another seizure in the emergency department and Abby was admitted. Her mother recalled, "If I hadn't watched my daughter and fought to get her help, she could have died!" Investigations revealed that Abby had an abnormal brain-wave pattern consistent with a seizure disorder, but not other medical problems.

Abby did not respond well to the seizure medication she was first prescribed, so there were several more trips to the emergency department, which were frightening for both mother and daughter. Abby's seizures were eventually controlled with a different medication and then became quite rare. Sleep deprivation, however, still provoked a seizure on occasion. Concerned for her daughter's well-being, Abby's mother initiated a very *regular sleep schedule* for her, ensured a *healthy diet and activity level*, and provided her medication with absolute consistency.

Factor Type	Risk Factors	Protective Factors	Impact on Child Development
Constitutional	*?*	*?*	• *Preexisting parental anxiety*
Direct effect on brain	• *Seizures* • *Anti-seizure medication*	• *Adequate sleep* • *Healthy lifestyle*	• *Mild cognitive impairment*
Indirect effects of illness Biological/ psychological (including somatic)	• *Child and parent anxious about seizure risk and school failure*		• *Academic problems* • *Family conflict*
Biological/ social	• *Heightened parental anxiety* • *Professional minimizes risk*	• *Organized family that adheres to medication* • *Tutor to help with academics*	• *Parental overprotection* • *Good seizure control*
Biological/ cultural or spiritual		• *Church support*	• *Reassurance* • *Religious coping*

FIGURE 3.3. Example of biological factors and their impact for Abby, a girl with a seizure disorder.

Unfortunately, the *medication affected Abby's cognitive abilities,* and she began to *struggle to complete her schoolwork. Afraid of failing at school,* she stayed up later and later to complete assignments and study for tests. When her mother discovered this pattern, she was alarmed and shouted at Abby, "What are you doing? Do you have a death wish?" She insisted on turning out the lights in Abby's room at 9 P.M., but Abby secretly continued her work using a flashlight. Eventually, this behavior provoked a seizure, and Abby confessed the truth. *The mother–daughter relationship deteriorated* after that point as Abby's *mother became increasingly anxious about seizures,* and Abby became increasingly anxious about school failure. As the fights with her mother increased, Abby's school performance declined further, as did her willingness to take the medication (which she now called "the dummy pills").

After several attempts to educate both mother and daughter about managing seizures and about the realistic level of risk they posed, it became clear that additional intervention was needed to reduce the anxiety and tension in this family. A *tutor* was found for Abby to help with the subjects she found most difficult, reducing her fear of failing at school. Abby's mother was encouraged to talk to *friends at church* about "taking a break" from her intense home life by allowing a friend to stay with her daughter sometimes. She found her church *community surprisingly accepting* of her daughter's plight, which she had previously not revealed because she had seen a child with seizures labeled "possessed" at the same church years earlier. *Praying together* with her friends for Abby's well-being reduced the mother's anxiety and made her feel supported. Gradually, both mother and daughter became less stressed and were able to enjoy each other's company again while *maintaining good control of Abby's seizures.*

This example illustrates how biological risk and protective factors, both those that affect the brain directly and those that are due to responses of the child and family to illness (i.e., indirect effects), can interact to cause or ameliorate psychological difficulties.

SOMATIC SYMPTOM AND RELATED DISORDERS

Somatic symptoms are physical symptoms that suggest a medical condition but are wholly or partially due to psychological factors. When these symptoms are persistent and interfere with the child's daily functioning, they are considered disorders (American Psychiatric Association, 2013). Somatic symptoms can, however, occur in the context of other disorders, and they may have a biological component. For example, anxious children often focus excessively on bodily sensations, so they may perceive pain intensely, resulting in muscle tension and anxiety about the cause of the pain, and muscle tension in turn increases their pain, resulting in further anxiety. This mechanism may account for the association between anxiety disorders and stomachaches or tension headaches. Similarly, children who suffer a viral illness associated with vomiting can subsequently develop symptoms of nausea that are due to anxiety about further vomiting. If that anxiety results in food restriction, these children are at risk for further medical problems and may be misdiagnosed as having eating disorders (Manassis & Kalman, 1990).

Somatic symptom and related disorders include somatic symptom disorder, conversion disorder, illness anxiety disorder, factitious disorder, and psychological factors affecting other medical conditions.

These disorders can sometimes co-occur with medical conditions. For example, children like Abby who have seizure disorders can sometimes exhibit pseudoseizures (i.e., seizure-like movements that are due to psychological factors) in response to stressful events.

Brief descriptions of the somatic symptom and related disorders follow (American Psychiatric Association, 2013). In somatic symptom disorder there are multiple symptoms not fully explained by a medical condition and not intentionally produced by the child. In conversion disorder, there is a motor or sensory deficit due to psychological factors, but this is not intentional and it is sometimes triggered by stress. For example, a child may suddenly appear unable to walk even though there is no muscular or neurological problem to explain this disability. A careful history will usually reveal a recent change or stress in the child's life (e.g., starting a new school, illness in a family member). Illness anxiety disorder is the fear of having a serious illness despite evidence to the contrary. In factitious disorder, symptoms are intentionally and falsely presented in oneself or others, usually in order to obtain attention from medical professionals. Psychological factors affecting other medical conditions are often seen in children with chronic medical illnesses. For example, children with diabetes may be noncompliant with some aspects of treatment for psychological reasons.

When symptoms are not intentionally produced, it is important to take an empathic, rehabilitative approach with affected children. They need professionals to accept their distressing experience as valid, while at the same time reassuring them that the symptoms are not due to a serious medical illness. Psychological factors that are contributing to the symptoms are sought and addressed. Concurrently, the child is encouraged to do as many daily activities as possible despite the symptoms until they gradually improve. Familiarity with the child and family's cultural background can also be helpful, as signs of physical illness legitimize mental illness in some cultures, and there are some culturally specific conditions that include somatic symptoms.

As previously mentioned, there is an intentional production of symptoms in factitious disorder, which is usually done in order to assume the sick role and garner attention from medical professionals. One variation on factitious disorder that is particularly relevant to child mental health has been termed "Munchausen-by-proxy" (Stirling, 2007). In this (fortunately rare) condition, a parent repeatedly brings his or her child to physicians for treatment of symptoms that are actually being created or fabricated by the parent, usually in order to elicit attention and sympathy from medical professionals. For example, a child is found to have blood in the urine, but the parent has actually contributed drops of his or her own blood to the sample. Because the child can suffer unnecessary medical investigations and sometimes other physical harm due to the parent's actions, this condition is considered a form of child abuse and should therefore be reported to child protective services.

When determining whether or not a child's medical symptoms could relate to psychological factors, some useful clues include:

- The child's symptoms are not consistent with what is known about human anatomy or physiology (e.g., glove-like numbness of the hand is not consistent with the distribution of nerves in this area).
- The child's symptoms are temporally related to a stressful event.
- The child's symptoms are not present during sleep.
- The child's symptoms vary by environment (e.g., child appears more symptomatic at home than at school or in hospital).
- There is an unusual response to medical intervention (e.g., improvement immediately upon taking medication, when it has not yet been absorbed by the body).

However, none of these clues is diagnostic and sometimes medical and somatic symptoms co-occur, so a thorough medical history and physical examination is still important to ensure the best outcome for the child.

DEVELOPMENTAL CONSIDERATIONS

The importance of various biological risk and protective factors can vary in relation to children's development. For example, for a 10-year-old like Abby school failure would seem very threatening, so the mild cognitive impairment resulting from her medication had a major impact on her life. If she had been a preschooler, mild cognitive impairment would have been far less significant. Similarly, medication-related weight gain may be much more upsetting to an adolescent (given that adolescents are often highly self-conscious) than to a younger child. Common concerns related to chronic illness and medical treatment are related to various age groups (preschoolers, school-age children, and adolescents) in Table 3.1. Each of these concerns can be found at all ages but is particularly salient for the age group it corresponds to in the table.

TABLE 3.1. Common Illness-Related Concerns at Different Ages

Age	Concern
Preschool age	• Magical wishes/fears about illness • Pain and illness seen as punishment • Fear of abandonment by family
School age	• Low independence/overprotection by family • Effect on competence/school performance • Fear of mutilation/loss of bodily integrity • Realistic view of death as permanent (starting at about age 8)
Adolescent	• Effect on body image • Effect on peer relationships • Effect on autonomy/rebelling against treatment • Concerns about effects on intimate relationships • Concerns about implications for long-term goals

Developmental delays, particularly cognitive delays, can have major psychological effects on children and families. As in other medical illnesses, the impact is different depending on whether problems are noticeable soon after birth or not until years later. Delays that are diagnosed early are usually more severe and so place greater practical burdens upon families. Mild intellectual delays or severe learning disabilities pose challenges too, though, and are sometimes difficult to detect. These children may present with anxiety or angry outbursts due to difficulty regulating emotions (called "executive function deficits"), low self-esteem due to school failure and/or feeling less competent than their peers, or family conflict related to any of these issues. Parents may be frustrated with the child's lack of progress and sometimes assume the child is willful or lazy. Alternatively, they may suspect that the child is delayed and feel anxious or blame themselves for his or her difficulties.

Diagnosis is complicated by the fact that assessing the child at one point in time does not necessarily reveal his or her developmental trajectory. For example, parents may report that a child is regressing (i.e., losing previously acquired skills) because the developmental gap between the child and his or her peers appears to be increasing. As shown in Figure 3.4, however, the child may actually be progressing but at a slower rate than his or her peers, or development may have slowed or reached a plateau. Families may struggle valiantly to help the child "catch up," but this goal may or may not be realistic, particularly in the case of children who are simply learning more slowly than

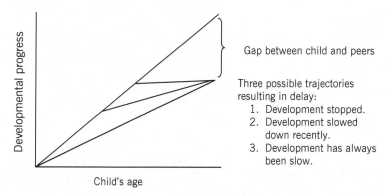

FIGURE 3.4. Developmental trajectories resulting in delay.

their peers. A grief reaction ensues as they begin to accept the child's intellectual disability and restricted long-term potential.

Social and community support, in addition to professional intervention, is essential to families of developmentally disabled children. North American culture tends to place a high value on individual achievement, often to the detriment of those who are "low achievers" by conventional standards. Consequently, many of these children are given unflattering labels related to their disabilities. As in Abby's case, supportive people or faith communities are often needed to make the child feel welcome and to appreciate his or her unique gifts.

As researchers understand more about brain development, however, a hopeful picture emerges. "Neuroplasticity" refers to the brain's continuing ability to change and adapt to its environment (reviewed in Doidge, 2007). Some aspects of brain development continue well into the 20s. For example, adolescents with limited insight and judgment can still develop these capacities at a later age. The frontal lobes of the brain, responsible for these abilities, continue to develop until age 25. Similarly, some cognitive deficits can be remediated with intensive practice. Such practice increases the connections between brain cells needed to perform particular cognitive skills, often improving the child's abilities beyond what was initially anticipated. If skills that used to be considered "hardwired" can change in this way, optimism regarding the more subtle psychological changes needed to improve the lives of our patients may also be warranted.

CHAPTER 4

Psychological Aspects
of the Formulation

In this chapter, we attempt to identify risk and protective factors that pertain to the child's developing inner world. Given the challenges of understanding what goes on in children's minds, the role of various theoretical models is discussed first. I then provide details regarding common cognitive and psychological challenges children face using ideas from two key theorists (Jean Piaget and Erik Erikson), with reference to other models that may provide a deeper understanding of particular challenges. In facing these obstacles, children eventually develop ways of coping (also called "defense mechanisms") that can sometimes produce symptoms, so these are briefly reviewed. Finally, recognizing that children's psychological development is inextricably linked with their environment, the concept of contextual influences on development is also introduced and illustrated with a case example. These influences are discussed in more detail in Chapters 5 and 6.

THEORETICAL CONSIDERATIONS

A common question that arises when discussing psychological development in children is "Which theory of psychological development do you subscribe to?" During the last century, dozens of different theories about children's psychological development have been proposed, and yet evidence for most of these theories is limited. There are several likely reasons for these disparate ideas. Young children cannot tell us what they think and feel, so we often infer thoughts and feelings based on their behavior, on what their parents tell us, and on our own conceptual models of how their psychology works. However, we cannot be sure that these inferences are accurate. Moreover, the nature of observation changes from one clinician to another: some prefer to observe children alone, others with their parents; some encourage children to play with toys in the office, others expect them to attend to questions or tasks. In short, we participate in the child's world even as we try to observe it, and the conclusions we draw from our observations are biased by our preconceived ideas about the child's mind. On the other hand, if no theoretical framework is used, some children's behaviors may seem to indicate the presence of psychopathology when in fact the behaviors are developmentally normal. Conversely, some behaviors may be seen as normative when in fact they are signs of psychological risk. For example, a 5-year-old child who expects her recently deceased parent to come home each night shows a normal grief reaction. Consistent with theories of cognitive development, 5-year-olds do not understand death as a permanent, irreversible reality. In contrast, a 15-year-old who loses a parent and expects him or her to reappear is clearly experiencing some sort of traumatic reaction, measured in part by the inappropriate developmental response. Theories of psychological development predict that a desire for autonomy from one's parents is normative in adolescence. Thus, theories can be a valuable guide to understanding which behaviors are developmentally appropriate at different ages and which ones are concerning.

Most theories of psychological development acknowledge that human beings must achieve certain broad psychological goals as they mature. These include developing an accurate and nuanced understanding of their environment, regulating their emotions (particularly negative emotions) so that these do not interfere with important tasks, and learning to relate to others in ways that are effective (i.e., both socially acceptable and consistent with their own needs). Positive psychologists (e.g., Seligman & Csikszentmihalyi, 2000) have recently added a capacity for optimism and positive emotion as an important goal, as past theories sometimes overemphasized reduction of distress or negative emotion.

Theories differ, however, in their descriptions of how these broad goals are achieved. One particular difference that often leads to debate is the presence or absence of certain stages of psychological development. Stage theorists often posit certain "critical periods" when a particular cognitive or psychological challenge must be faced if sub-sequent development is to follow a normal course. Sometimes experi-mental evidence supports or partially supports such stages and criti-cal periods, and sometimes it does not. For example, in early infancy the need to develop a close, trusting bond (as postulated in Erikson's developmental stages [Erikson, 1959]) has been supported extensively by experiments carried out by attachment researchers (Rutter, 1995). Infants who do not develop a secure attachment are at increased risk for many adverse developmental outcomes (Rutter, 1995). However, these experiments have not shown that infants with insecure attach-ments are irreparably damaged. Over time, there are further opportu-nities to address the issue of trust and mistrust in relationships, so that by adulthood there are people who were clearly abused or neglected in early childhood but have developed so-called "earned secure" attach-ment styles (Bretherton & Munholland, 1999). In this case, early infancy is a *relative* critical period, as it is easiest to develop a capacity for trust at this time, but it is still possible to develop that capacity later.

In case formulation, it may be useful to think about developmen-tal challenges proposed by stage theorists with an understanding that each challenge is not necessarily limited to a particular age but may resurface at various times as children mature. The stages proposed may still provide some guidance as to a challenge that might be more or less significant for a child at a given time. For example, I have seen some parents express concern that their preschool children will develop "an unhealthy identity as a mental patient" if given a psychiatric diagnosis. I usually reassure them that identity formation will not be consolidated until much later in development (Erikson, 1959), and that children are more likely to be concerned about missing out on something fun because they have to go to therapy. Nevertheless, one shouldn't assume that just because a child is of a particular age he or she is in a particular stage or struggling with a particular challenge.

COGNITIVE DEVELOPMENT

Jean Piaget was a Swiss developmental psychologist who described stages of cognitive development in the 1940s, largely based on observa-tions of his own three children, that are still relevant today (reviewed in Piaget, 1977). The exact time course of these stages has been found to vary a great deal, particularly in youth with developmental disabili-ties (Williams, 1996), and the most advanced stage (formal operations) is not reached by all adults (Berk, 2007). The sequence of cognitive abilities he described, however, provides an elegant description of how humans learn to perceive and think about their world and themselves.

Understanding this development of cognitive abilities is relevant to mental health in several ways. Parents who have an understanding of their children's cognitive abilities tend to have more realistic expectations of their behavior, often reflected in more effective behavior management strategies and fewer family conflicts. Child therapists who understand cognition are more likely to be able to better tailor their therapeutic techniques to the child's capacity to understand. This issue is particularly relevant to therapies that emphasize cognition, such as cognitive-behavioral therapy (CBT). In case formulation, it is important to understand how the presence or absence of certain cognitive abilities can affect the psychological goals children struggle to achieve, that is, the ability to regulate emotions, to relate successfully to others, and to maintain a capacity for optimism.

Piaget described children's progression through various cognitive stages as resulting from two processes: assimilation and accommodation (Piaget, 1977). In assimilation, the child understands a new object or stimulus in terms of an existing mental structure. In accommodation, the child encounters an object or stimulus that is difficult to reconcile with existing mental structures, so cognitive reorganization takes place in order to adapt to (or "accommodate") that stimulus. Thus, rather than passively receiving knowledge, the child continually and actively interacts with the environment to construct and reconstruct a mental picture of reality.

The four stages Piaget described are (in developmental order): the sensorimotor stage, the preoperational stage, the concrete operational stage, and the formal operational stage. In children whose development progresses at an average rate, these stages roughly correspond to infancy, the preschool years, early school age, and adolescence. During the sensorimotor stage, infants experience the world through the five senses. They are self-focused, and so cannot perceive the world from others' points of view. They gradually develop the ability to understand that objects continue to exist when they cannot see them. For example, an infant at the beginning of this stage cannot understand a "shell game" where an object is covered by a shell, the shell is moved, and a second shell is put in its place. The infant will look for the object in the location where it was last seen (i.e., under the second shell). By the end of the sensorimotor stage, the infant will find the object under the correct shell even though the shell's location has changed.

In the preoperational stage, language, memory, and imagination develop. Thinking is intuitive and sometimes magical in nature. Children at this age often engage in wishful thinking and may not clearly distinguish what is wished for from what is realistically possible. Their concept of time is vague and they do not plan ahead. Another cognitive limitation is the need to attend to one dimension at a time, described as a "failure to conserve." For example, the child cannot understand that a tall, thin glass may contain the same amount of milk as a short, wide glass.

In the concrete operational stage, children become able to see the world from others' points of view. This does not necessarily imply empathy for others' feelings, but rather an intellectual understanding of others' perspective. For instance, a child may understand that she is a girl, her mother's daughter (understanding the mother's perspective), and her brother's sister (understanding the brother's perspective). The child thinks more realistically, no longer struggles to attend to more than one dimension at a time, and starts to manipulate symbols that relate to concrete objects, allowing him, for example, to begin to grasp mathematics. However, abstract concepts and hypothetical thinking are still challenging.

In the formal operational stage, abstract and hypothetical thinking are fully developed. The ability to formulate and test hypotheses allows the adolescent to engage in scientific inquiry. The capacity for manipulating ideas that are abstract (i.e., independent of concrete objects) allows for introspection and philosophical reasoning. The teenager can also consider multiple courses of action and their attendant risks and benefits, allowing for independent problem solving, planning, and logical decision making. There is still a tendency for adolescents to overemphasize their uniqueness and invincibility (sometimes called the "personal fable") and the scrutiny of others (sometimes called the "imaginary audience"). Yet, sophisticated reasoning is possible at this stage.

This understanding of cognitive development leads to some common clinical and psychological implications that are helpful for parents and practitioners to keep in mind. They can also contribute to successful case formulation when cognitive factors are at play. A few implications often encountered in clinical practice include:

- Children are often mistakenly accused of being "manipulative" (i.e., deliberately planning to achieve their goals or meet their emotional needs through self-serving, devious strategies) at ages when this cognitive ability simply does not exist. Preadolescent children are highly dependent on adults to help them develop effective ways to regulate their feelings and meet their emotional needs. Few are able to "manipulate" others.

- Children can deal with serious issues (e.g., a death or life-threatening illness in the family; an impending divorce) if these issues are explained in a supportive, age-appropriate fashion. In the absence of an explanation, preschoolers in particular often imagine something even worse than what has really happened. Repeated explanations may be needed, however, as the child's cognitive understanding of the situation changes year by year (as in the example of the bereaved 5-year-old described at the beginning of this chapter).

- Young children's short time perspective can make it difficult for them to delay gratification (e.g., wait until after dinner for the cookie) or be reassured by promises of better times to come.

- When children are taught to share and cannot learn to do so, this behavior may sometimes reflect a young child's cognitive inability to conserve, rather than selfish behavior (as in the "glass of milk" example above).

- Children of all ages are capable of empathy but understand the concept differently. Thus, the preschooler who sees a peer crying about a lost toy may intuitively sense her sadness and cry along; the school-age child may understand that his friend is struggling with the loss of a cherished possession and offer comfort; the adolescent is more likely able to both cognitively and emotionally understand the loss. Moreover, these older children may also have the capacity to consider different options to help their friend deal with the challenges of the loss. Thus, expecting young children to "put themselves in the other person's shoes" is not always realistic.

- Problem-solving skills require adult guidance in preadolescents, and sometimes in adolescents too (recall that not all adolescents achieve formal operational reasoning). Providing choices about day-to-day events (e.g., a chance to choose a type of sandwich to have for lunch or choose a destination for a family outing) and encouraging children to evaluate the pros and cons of different options are nice stepping-stones toward this ability (see Manassis, 2012, for more details).

- The capacity to "think about thinking" (metacognition—the final executive function to be acquired) is rarely developed in preadolescents, so this skill may need to be practiced before they can use it in psychotherapy. Even with practice, children's ability to do this may be limited. Therefore, therapists must sometimes provide concrete reminders or encourage children to use the same helpful thoughts repeatedly (e.g., substituting the same reassuring thoughts in place of anxious thoughts when treating anxiety) when using cognitive or cognitive-behavioral approaches.

- The sophisticated reasoning of adolescents does not always coexist with a sophisticated social or emotional understanding. Social judgment and emotion regulation continue to develop well into young adulthood. Therefore, even highly intelligent adolescents often need practice in these areas. For example, many adolescents understand that their actions have potentially serious consequences but tell themselves, "It won't happen to me." This adolescent myth of personal invincibility can, unfortunately, have tragic results.

PSYCHOLOGICAL DEVELOPMENT

Erik Erikson was a developmental psychologist of the late 20th century who wrote extensively about psychological development across the life span. He proposed eight stages that began in infancy and continued until death and were defined by specific psychological challenges (Erikson, 1959). Only the first six of Erikson's challenges are described here, as the last two are more relevant to adult than child or adolescent development. Although there are limitations to all stage-based theories, as we have just discussed, the challenges Erikson described are so basic to the human condition that they are relevant regardless of one's theoretical orientation. Some theorists, however, explore a particular challenge in greater depth than others do. Therefore, when discussing each challenge, I also cite those theorists who may provide a deeper understanding of that particular challenge. Table 4.1 illustrates the six child and adolescent developmental challenges and also the familial and social supports that may be needed to facilitate a child's successful mastery of each challenge.

Trust versus Mistrust

Erikson postulated that the first challenge was faced in infancy and consisted of developing a sense that caretakers are trustworthy. John Bowlby's attachment theory examines this challenge in more detail and is now supported by a substantial evidence base (reviewed in

TABLE 4.1. Erikson's Child and Adolescent Developmental Challenges and Supports Needed

Challenge	Developmental change	Familial and social support
Trust versus mistrust	• Parent–child attachment security • Physiological regulation facilitated by attachment relationship • Beginnings of exploration (once mobile)	• Support of marital partner, extended family, community • Societal support of new mothers • Family safety and financial stability • Parental knowledge re: parenting and temperament variation
Autonomy versus shame and doubt	• Recognition of self as a separate being • Feeling acceptable as an individual • Further exploration • Beginnings of self-regulation	• Parental playfulness and respect for boundaries • Acceptability of child in this family/culture • Encouragement of exploration • Praise for toileting efforts • High-quality day care
Initiative versus guilt	• Curiosity • Delight in one's own actions • Developing healthy limits to one's actions (e.g., delaying gratification) • Sibling relationships • Social contact outside the family	• Developmentally informed and consistent parental discipline practices • Encouragement of independent activity • Attention to emerging interests and aptitudes • Facilitating peer contact
Industry versus inferiority	• Managing school (e.g., punctuality, sitting and listening, learning, getting along) • Activities outside school • Friendships • Responsibilities at home • Being proud of achievement without necessarily "winning"	• Developmentally informed and consistent school and home expectations • Home and school communication and support for positive peer relationships • Healthy cultural and community activities • Culture values effort and cooperation, not just success in competition
Identity versus role diffusion	• Negotiating autonomy from parents and eventually peers • Developing skills and interests	• Parents' and schools' ability to gradually increase freedom with responsibility, tolerate benign experimentation, set limits when needed, support individuation and goal setting

(continued)

TABLE 4.1. (continued)

Challenge	Developmental change	Familial and social support
	• Comfort with gender and sexual orientation • Developing long-term goals	• Prosocial teen activities and role models • Cultural/spiritual identity rituals
Intimacy versus isolation	• Risking close relationships that entail respect, vulnerability, and interdependence • Eventual commitment to a partner • Often a chance to revisit attachment issues	• Role models of healthy relationships at home, outside home, and in the media • Continuing friendships and supportive family relationships when in intimate relationship • Cultural/spiritual supports for long-term commitments and families

Bretherton, 1992; Rutter, 1995). Optimal attachment (termed "secure attachment") occurs when the infant comes to expect a consistent and sensitive response from the parent when distressed. As the infant begins to rely on the parent, he or she protests when briefly separated from the parent and calms quickly when reunited with the parent (an experimental attachment measure termed the "Strange Situation procedure"). Once securely attached, the infant is no longer constantly focused on the parent's availability and so becomes free to explore his or her surroundings. Eventually, the secure relationship with the parent creates a template (also termed "cognitive schema" or "internal working model"; Bretherton & Munholland, 1999) for other close relationships, influencing the developing child's expectations of others and of himself or herself in relation to others in the long run. Secure attachment has been linked to numerous positive mental health outcomes and has also been found beneficial in regulating various aspects of infant physiology (Fox & Hane, 2008). Common suboptimal attachment patterns include avoidant attachment, whereby the infant learns to minimize signs of distress as these are not welcome by the parent; ambivalent attachment, whereby the infant learns to amplify signs of distress to gain the attention of an inconsistently responsive parent; and disorganized attachment, whereby the parent (sometimes as a result of psychiatric problems) behaves unpredictably in response to infant distress. Infants with disorganized attachment sometimes develop either controlling or caregiving behaviors toward the parent. It is helpful to keep these possibilities in mind when constructing case formulations for children who show emotion regulation difficulties and/or families with emotionally distant or emotionally conflicted relationship patterns.

Attachment theory is sometimes misunderstood as a "parent-blaming" theory, but this is not its intention. Rather, attachment patterns seem to cross the generations, and most parents with insecure attachments to their infants grew up in insecure relationships with their parents as well. Moreover, unless parents become aware of their typical attachment style and work with a therapist to modify it, most are unaware of their own attachment behaviors and perceive themselves as simply doing "what comes naturally" in parenting. Furthermore, the most disrupted attachment pattern (disorganized attachment) is often linked to parental psychopathology, parental traumatic experiences, or grief. Thus, it may result from factors that are largely outside the parent's control.

As shown in Table 4.1, secure attachment may also depend on having good supports for new mothers and their babies. Supportive spouses, friends, and members of the extended family and the parents' community supports can all reduce maternal stress and contribute to healthy mother–infant relationships. Adequate parental leave, good nutrition and financial stability, and living in a safe neighborhood are important too and speak to the need for child- and family-friendly social policies. Education about normal development and expected variations in temperament can relieve both anxiety and frustration in new parents. Attachment-focused interventions have also shown some success in high-risk families (Berlin, Zeanah, & Lieberman, 2008).

Autonomy versus Shame and Doubt

Erikson's second challenge pertains to the development of autonomy. However, since it corresponds to the toddler years developmentally, it is not intended to be synonymous with children becoming fully independent. Instead, Erikson acknowledges the developing child's increasing recognition of himself or herself as an autonomous individual, separate and different from the parent, and acceptable as such. Shame and doubt are experienced when the child is made to feel different in a negative way as, for example, when a parent reacts with disgust to a toddler's unsuccessful attempt to use the toilet rather than praising successful ones.

Often, however, descriptions of this challenge have focused excessively on harsh toileting practices and neglected the broader definition of shame as a negative self-appraisal based on others' evaluation (Lewis, 1971). Shaming behaviors such as ridiculing a child or failing to respect interpersonal boundaries are obvious, but more subtle forms exist as well and can be significant developmentally. Families in which children are repeatedly made to feel unacceptable for various reasons (e.g., having a different temperament from other family members; being the "wrong" gender), in which attempts at individual expression are repeatedly discouraged, or in which children are expected to closely mirror their parents' behavior (regardless of how they feel) can also generate shame.

D. W. Winnicott (1965) described children who developed a "false self" of polite and well-mannered behavior, usually to please their parents, but were not able to feel spontaneous or happy because they were not being authentic or true to themselves. By contrast, he described "good-enough" parents as usually being emotionally attuned to their children's needs (though not perfectly so), thus allowing children to express themselves more freely without fearing shame or parental disapproval. Such parents also have the capacity to enjoy their children's unique characteristics, to be playful, and to see things from the child's point of view.

Nevertheless, mastering this challenge is not entirely attributable to parenting style. First, "good enough" parenting is clearly easier in some circumstances than others. Parents who are in supportive relationships, do not have overly stressful jobs, and are not struggling to obtain the basic necessities of life are more likely to engage in positive parenting behaviors. The arrival of another child (when siblings are closely spaced) can also strain parents' ability to be adequately attuned to their children. Second, most toddlers in North America have nonparental caregivers at least some of the time, and many attend day care centers. High-quality, developmentally sensitive child care is crucial in promoting children's healthy emotional development. For example, some day care centers will threaten to expel children who are not toilet trained by a particular age, blaming the parents for this perceived deficit or shaming the child in front of his or her peers. Such policies are clearly not conducive to healthy emotional development in the toddler.

Initiative versus Guilt

Erikson's third challenge is thought to be most relevant in preschoolers. This challenge concerns what the child does, rather than who the child is. Children explore, begin to create (e.g., painting or building with blocks), and learn to look after some of their daily needs (e.g., dressing or using utensils to eat). They also take "initiative" in fighting with siblings, sneaking treats when not allowed, not sharing their toys with peers, and other minor misbehavior. Thus, this challenge is as much about developing healthy self-control as it is about developing independent initiative.

Parents and other adults in the child's life have the opportunity to attend to and foster children's curiosity, independence, and interests. For example, the first time the child decides to get a glass of juice from the refrigerator independently, the result is likely to be a rather messy kitchen. Some parents will react very negatively to the mess, without praising or even acknowledging the independent effort. Other parents will say something encouraging such as "Good try! Here's how you pour it. I know you'll get it with practice. Now, let's clean up." The latter response is much more likely to foster initiative and independence. Facilitating "playdates" and other forms of social contact with peers can also foster independence and help develop social skills.

Parents and other adults in the child's life must also come to some agreement as to what constitutes acceptable and unacceptable behavior, and how to manage the latter. Volumes have been written on this subject, but most agree that calm, consistent responses to misbehavior that are not overly harsh reduce the misbehavior over time (Brestan & Eyberg, 1998). From the child's point of view, such responses clearly indicate that the behavior is not acceptable but the child still is acceptable to the adult. This message increases the chances that the behavioral standard that has been enforced is eventually internalized by the child, fostering a healthy self-discipline. Similarly, overly harsh or overly critical discipline can foster excessive self-criticism and unrealistic personal standards, and inconsistent or overly emotional discipline can foster poor self-control.

Since Freud's original description of the id, ego, and superego (1933), numerous theorists have tried to describe the tension humans experience between wanting to gratify their impulses (the pleasure-seeking "id" in Freud's terms) and behaving in ways that are considered respectable (the "superego" in Freud's terms). The need to manage these competing desires by developing a strong "ego" (in other words, a psychological manager of this conflict) has received particular emphasis. Theories aside, many children from preschool age onward who are overly self-critical or overly impulsive will identify this tension. "I have an angel on one shoulder and a devil on the other" is one metaphor they sometimes use, perhaps because it shows up occasionally in popular cartoons. "I'm like a guy in a chariot with two horses to steer" is another one a young boy described to me once in psychotherapy.

An understanding of this common dilemma can often aid in formulation. For example, I recently saw a young man of about 15 who had suffered from social anxiety in the past (now in remission) and was now experiencing a new onset of panic attacks after being offered marijuana by a friend. He refused the marijuana but went through daily panic attacks afterwards. After exploring the story in more detail, it became clear that he was a deeply religious teen, and he and his family considered all drug use abhorrent to God. Nevertheless, when offered the marijuana he had been tempted to take it, despite his beliefs. When describing his panic attacks, he said he feared losing control of himself and his life and never being able to regain it. When asked what would have happened if he had taken the marijuana, he described it in very similar terms. Making this connection seemed to be helpful to him and led to a discussion of his high personal standards and how it is normal for most people to feel "tempted" on occasion. His panic attacks resolved without further intervention.

Industry versus Inferiority

This is a challenge that Erikson describes in relation to school-age children. At this age, children focus on comparing themselves to others in various arenas of life. Academic comparisons occur regularly at school. Athletic ability, physical appearance, character strengths, social acceptance, and the ability to form close friendships can also be sources of comparison though (Harter, 1998), and may contribute to children's sense of self-worth and esteem. Concerns about inferiority and self-esteem have been discussed by numerous theorists beginning with Alfred Adler, a contemporary of Freud who advocated a democratic approach to parenting to avoid generating feelings of inferiority in children (Adler, 1964).

As indicated in Table 4.1, success at school involves a number of component skills, and difficulty with any of these skills can undermine a child's academic achievement. These skills can include cognitive skills needed to learn, social skills, and the ability to organize oneself and regulate one's emotions (so-called "executive functions"). Strengths in other areas can sometimes offset the negative effect of academic failure on self-esteem, however. Good communication between parents and schools is essential to supporting children's academic progress. Communication is particularly important when the child does not fall within the academic average, either because of an intellectual or learning disability or because of high intellectual ability (i.e., gifted children often struggle in traditional school settings as well). Parental support is less crucial in forming and maintaining friendships at school age than at younger ages but can still be needed when difficulties occur (e.g., if a child is severely teased or bullied). Parents can also facilitate access to activities outside of school where children can develop their strengths and/or gain an understanding of their heritage.

Emotional and behavioral problems in children often come to clinical attention in the early school years. Usually, this is not due to the new onset of problems but rather to the fact that the expectations of children's behavior increase at this age. At school, children are expected to do progressively larger quantities of work with progressively less guidance and direction from the teacher. At home, children are often expected to contribute to the housework by doing a few chores, to independently take care of basic hygiene, and to develop regular homework routines. Some parents have additional expectations in relation to the family's cultural background, and these may differ for boys and girls. For example, girls may be expected to help with younger siblings or to do a greater share of household chores than boys in some cultures. On the other hand, academic expectations may be higher for boys than for girls in some cultures. When familial expectations differ dramatically from those of the local culture, children may feel torn between obedience to their families and successful adaptation to the environment outside the home.

In North America, stresses related to this developmental challenge may be heightened by a cultural emphasis on individualism and competition. Individuals who work hard and succeed with apparently little assistance from others are generally admired, and the support they received from others and from favorable circumstances is minimized. Winners in competitive professional sports become celebrities. By contrast, contributing one's best effort to a group project or engaging in recreational sports for good health and enjoyment garners less attention. As a result, children sometimes have difficulty feeling positive about their efforts when they are not linked to winning a prize or when they have accepted others' help in order to succeed.

Identity versus Role Diffusion

Erikson describes the consolidation of identity (in comparison to "role diffusion," in which identity is not successfully established) as the major challenge of adolescence. Several tasks are involved, including developing increasing autonomy from the family of origin, comfort with various aspects of the self, developing long-term goals, and developing a sense of "fitting in" with the rest of the world. Erikson himself wrote extensively about the challenges of identity development, as his culturally mixed heritage left him feeling like an outsider in his youth. Other theorists have emphasized different identity-related tasks, for example, referring to adolescence as the "second separation–individuation" (Blos, 1979) or (more recently) describing the challenge of reconciling a nonheterosexual orientation with a healthy sense of self (Stronski & Remafedi, 1998).

One important developmental principle to bear in mind is that adolescent identity formation can be thought of as a culmination of previous developmental tasks. Masten and Coatsworth (1998) emphasize that the internal resources the adolescent has available for resolving the developmental tasks of adolescence depend on the resolution of developmental tasks in childhood. For example, a young woman whose attempts at self-expression have been invalidated in early childhood may cope by behaving in an overly agreeable manner with her parents. Upon developing abstract reasoning abilities in adolescence, however, she begins to formulate worldviews that conflict with those of her parents. However, since the parent–child relationship has always been predicated upon her agreeable behavior, she cannot express her views without risking a sudden rupture of that relationship. Gradual striving toward autonomy is therefore difficult, and this difficulty may result in clinical symptoms. Similarly, difficulties with trust, initiative, self-discipline, industry, and self-esteem can all reemerge in the context of adolescent identity struggles. From a more positive perspective, healthy childhood development provides the foundation for healthy adolescent development.

On the other hand, Cicchetti and Rogosch (2002) have written about the opportunities for developmental reorganization that exist in adolescence, as the balance of risk and protective processes can shift dramatically at this age. One example from my practice is that of a young man who chronically avoided school and struggled with his parents and various mental health agencies for years around this issue. Finally, he reached an age when school attendance was no longer mandatory, so his parents gave him the option of either getting a job or returning to school. As a high school dropout, one of the few jobs he was qualified to do was stocking shelves at the local supermarket. After several months of stocking shelves and dealing with his rather unpleasant coworkers and boss, he enthusiastically returned to school.

One challenge for parents of adolescents is the oscillating nature of autonomy development. *Get Out of My Life, but First Could You Drive Me and Cheryl to the Mall?* (Wolf, 2002) was a popular book on the subject. It highlights the tendency for adolescents to move to and fro between accepting and rejecting parental norms and values, often depending on their own needs at the time. Identification with peer values is common in early and mid-adolescence. Older adolescents eventually learn to "agree to disagree" with parents and peers alike, as they become more comfortable with their own personal values. Wise parents tolerate the inconsistencies of adolescent striving for autonomy with patience, support, and a bit of humor. In addition, privileges and freedoms the young person enjoys are gradually increased as he or she demonstrates the ability to handle them responsibly. Some benign experimentation is tolerated (e.g., with clothing styles, music, and food preferences), but limits are set when needed to ensure safety and reduce the chances of highly adverse consequences (e.g., incarceration or teen pregnancy). When parents and teens maintain good communication, parents may also be able to support adolescents in setting long-term goals and finding their "niche" in relation to the rest of the world.

For teens from families that have recently immigrated to North America, differences between familial norms for behavior and those of the predominant culture may be accentuated. Adolescent attempts to establish autonomy from their families may be punished severely, or carried out in secret. For example, a female teen growing up in an area of a North American city where the population is predominantly of southern European origin might struggle with cultural prohibitions against dating. Such tensions are not necessarily reflective of particular ethnic groups, but rather of the degree of acculturation of families within those groups. Inquiring about comfort with the local culture is therefore an important aspect of assessment in these families.

Given the adolescent tendency to identify with peers, supportive peer groups and activities can affect identity development in a positive way. For example, teen clubs that focus on environmental or social justice issues are found in many schools, as are athletic teams and student councils or other leadership opportunities. Healthy teen role models in the media can also exert a positive influence, although media influences can also be detrimental (e.g., identifying with unrealistically thin models can increase the risk of eating disorders). Spiritual or cultural rituals that mark a new stage or life or of community membership (e.g., confirmation, bar/bat mitzvah) can also encourage a more "grown-up" identity for some teens, although others experience them as a source of pressure to conform to family values.

Intimacy versus Isolation

According to Erikson, the capacity for intimate relationships (vs. isolating oneself from these) develops in young adulthood, but intimacy issues commonly begin to present in adolescence and so merit some discussion here. The capacity for intimate relationships includes but is not limited to healthy sexual relationships. Intimacy, broadly speaking, includes all aspects of relationships that involve interdependence. It requires trust, mutual respect, and comfort with one's own vulnerability (as, for example, when risking a partner's disapproval by discussing something unpleasant). Some intimate relationships eventually become long-term, committed partnerships.

The childhood challenge that is most closely linked to the capacity for intimacy is that of trust versus mistrust. Consequently, patterns of attachment that were established with parents in infancy sometimes reemerge in intimate relationships (Hazan & Shaver, 1987). Mental models (or assumptions) with respect to attachment figures are often transferred onto intimate partners. For example, someone with a history of an inconsistently available attachment figure may be insecure about his or her partner's availability, resulting in overly dependent behavior. Someone whose parents discouraged the expression of negative emotion may have difficulty communicating negative feelings with an intimate partner.

Rejection by an intimate partner is a common trigger for distress and psychiatric symptoms in adolescents. It may be particularly devastating for those with insecure attachment histories, as these teens often wish for relationships that will repair past hurts experienced in their family of origin, even if they are not consciously aware of this wish. In teens who are still struggling with identity issues, loss of an intimate relationship may also result in questions about their own self-worth. The psychological crisis of coping with relationship loss, however, can also be an opportunity to engage the adolescent in treatment that addresses his or her difficulties related to attachment and intimacy.

Adolescents who are involved in intimate relationships are sometimes overly focused on their partner to the exclusion of other supportive people in their lives. Given the potential consequences of relationship loss mentioned above, this strategy is risky. Continuing friendships outside the relationship and continuing to nurture positive family relationships should therefore be encouraged. Friends and family members can also provide important role models of healthy, interdependent relationships. Unfortunately, such role models are often scarce in the popular media.

COPING AND DEFENSIVE STYLES

Many psychiatric symptoms represent maladaptive ways of coping with distress, so understanding child coping at different ages can help us understand symptom formation when constructing a case formulation. Interestingly, a number of coping strategies are also considered "defense mechanisms" by some writers. The former term has a much more positive connotation than the latter, but the difference is largely philosophical. Both coping strategies and defense mechanisms serve the same function: to modulate negative, distressing emotions.

In infancy, children's options when distressed are limited. Infants are almost totally dependent on seeking support from their caregivers. As children become mobile, additional behavioral options emerge. These include acting-out behaviors (e.g., temper tantrums), avoiding or withdrawing from the distressing situation, and remaining in the distressing situation but limiting the expression of emotion. With increased cognitive development, children can begin to distract themselves from distressing circumstances, positively reappraise distressing circumstances, and engage in problem solving to address the source of the distress. Thus, as children mature their coping strategies become more varied and sophisticated.

In adults, appraisal- and problem-focused coping strategies are generally considered more adaptive than emotion-focused strategies (Taylor, 2006). However, as young children's cognitive abilities may limit their capacity for reappraisal and their dependence on the environment may limit their problem-solving options, strategies should probably only be considered maladaptive in childhood when they clearly interfere with important developmental tasks (e.g., chronic avoidance of social situations interfering with the development of friendships and social skills). Other authors have emphasized the importance of a wide repertoire of coping strategies (Lazarus & Folkman, 1984). That is, it may be more beneficial to help children develop multiple, alternative coping strategies than to label some strategies as particularly adaptive or particularly maladaptive.

As mentioned earlier, defenses overlap considerably with coping strategies. Dozens of defenses have been described in the literature, but George Vaillant (1992) classified common ones into four levels: pathological, immature, neurotic, and adaptive. Only the first level (pathological) is regularly associated with psychopathology. Defenses at this level include projection (attributing one's own shortcomings to others), conversion (e.g., blindness or paralysis that has no medical cause; see Chapter 3), denial of reality to meet one's own needs, distortion of reality to meet one's own needs, and splitting (a tendency to see others as either entirely good or entirely evil). As with coping strategies, however, defenses need to be viewed in the context of development. It is not unusual for preschoolers, for example, to deny or distort reality given that preoperational thought is not entirely realistic.

When considering coping strategies or defenses in case formulation, it is often helpful to look for maladaptive patterns of behavior that the child seems unable to change. These often represent a maladaptive coping strategy or defense. Sometimes, parents are reinforcing the pattern, often without meaning to. For example, sometimes children engage in excessive support seeking from caregivers even when this is no longer necessary. A school-age child might still ask a parent to assist with cutting up food or dressing in the morning. In this case, parental attention is emotionally soothing to the child but interferes with the age-appropriate development of independent self-care. A parent who enjoys nurturing the child may indulge his or her requests, inadvertently hampering this important developmental step. Children who almost always respond to distress by acting out or by avoiding upsetting situations may also be "caught" in a maladaptive coping pattern.

Fortunately, the younger the child the more malleable his or her coping and defensive strategies tend to be. For example, in CBT children regularly expand their repertoire of coping strategies significantly in a matter of 3 or 4 months. It is not until adolescence that coping and defensive strategies start to become entrenched. The DSM-5 (American Psychiatric Association, 2013) recognizes this phenomenon by not permitting some personality disorder diagnoses (which reflect chronic use of maladaptive strategies) in children under the age of 18. With professional help, even adults can still change their habitual patterns of thought and behavior, but doing so requires more effort than in childhood.

THE CONTEXT OF CHILDREN'S PSYCHOLOGICAL DEVELOPMENT

Figure 4.1 illustrates some key points about the context of children's psychological development. These points will be briefly discussed here, and a more detailed discussion of environmental factors follows in Chapters 5 and 6. In Figure 4.1, the child's mind is considered to be at the core of psychological development, surrounded by family influences and by the larger social environment. At birth, constitutional factors largely dictate the child's state of mind, but almost immediately parental and family influences come into play. These influences remain salient throughout development, although the larger social environment assumes increasing importance as the child moves toward maturity (as represented by the increased width of the social environment trapezoids in the figure at maturity). The arrows represent (respectively) the reciprocal interactions between the child's mind and the family, between the family and the larger social environment, and between the child's mind and the larger social environment. Notice that the latter becomes more substantial as the child matures. In young children, however, almost all interaction with the larger social environment is mediated by the family. Thus, the family not only influences the child directly, but indirectly through the willingness to facilitate (or not facilitate) access to other social influences. In families that are warm and supportive of the child's development, limited access to the larger social environment may not have many adverse results. In highly problematic families, it can be disastrous.

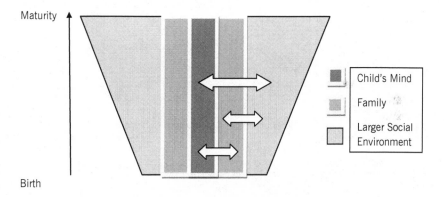

FIGURE 4.1. The context for psychological development.

Some of these effects will now be illustrated with a case example, summarized in Figure 4.2. Figure 4.3, which can be photocopied for clinical use, is provided to allow clinicians to summarize cognitive challenges, psychological challenges, relevant coping styles, and relevant biological and contextual factors, and their impact when formulating child psychological development. Notice in the following story how the factors recorded in the table are placed in chronological order and then related to each other to create a hypothetical description of how Serena's difficulties could have developed. Key factors from the table are *italicized* in the example below.

Factor Type	Risk Factors	Protective Factors	Impact
Cognitive challenge	• *School and parents expect her to demonstrate conceptual reasoning*		• *Failure to keep up at school adversely affects self-esteem*
Psychological challenge	• *Academic achievement is needed for self-esteem* • *Development of self-control and trust still lagging*	• *Anxiety limits oppositionality at school*	• *Reduced motivation to succeed at school and control behavior* • *Mistrust of authority figures reduces cooperation*
Coping style	• *Child seeks attention through acting out* • *Family isolates and terminates therapies*	• *Engages with therapist, but superficially*	• *Habitual negative interaction* • *Failed attempts at therapy*
Biological and contextual factors	• *Difficult temperament* • *Language-based learning disability* • *Possible ADHD* • *High-conflict family* • *Inconsistent behavior management* • *Probable attachment insecurity*	• *Socially adept* • *School culture is helpful rather than punitive*	• *Learned helplessness regarding academics* • *Difficulty regulating all emotions* • *Lack of structure and consistency worsens behavior and anxiety* • *Popular among peers*

FIGURE 4.2. Example of psychological factors and their impact for Serena, a girl with severe oppositionality.

Factor Type	Risk Factors	Protective Factors	Impact
Cognitive challenge			
Psychological challenge			
Coping style			
Biological and contextual factors			

FIGURE 4.3. Psychological factors and their impact on development.

Case Example: Serena

Serena was an 11-year-old girl who was an only child born into an affluent but *highly conflicted, divorced family.* When assessed in a psychiatric clinic, she met criteria for oppositional defiant disorder, ADHD, and generalized anxiety disorder. Although not meeting criteria for depression, she reported matter-of-factly, "I don't see things getting any better." She had recently been hospitalized following a violent outburst in which her mother was injured. The consultation request read "query bipolar child."

Serena was described as always having had a *difficult temperament.* She was very emotionally intense, persistent when she wanted something, and "destroyed anything she couldn't figure out right away." Serena's mother suffered from postpartum depression and acknowledged having *difficulty bonding with her child.* She also reported *domestic violence* at the hands of her ex-husband, although he never harmed Serena. Serena's parents separated when Serena was 3 years old, but court proceedings concerning custody and child support continued for several years afterwards and she continued to see both parents. Serena's parents still argued daily on the phone.

Serena's misbehavior was reportedly a lifelong problem, although it had intensified after the parental separation. There was no fluctuation in the level of misbehavior, nor any clear variability in mood. *When Serena misbehaved, her mother tried to reason with her and "teach her" how to behave better, often resulting in arguments. Her father, on the other hand, would either lock her in her room until she settled down or "bribe her" with a treat* so she would behave better. Neither parent had found an approach that was effective.

Upon starting school, Serena lagged behind academically and was found to have a *language-based learning disability as well as ADHD.* She mistrusted and felt intimidated by teachers, however, and so *limited her misbehavior at school.* She soon considered herself "stupid" and began smoking in the bathroom with older girls. She was frustrated by her learning difficulty and soon began avoiding schoolwork before even attempting it. However, she often made jokes in class, and so was quite *popular* among her peers. After meeting her highly argumentative parents, *her schoolteachers also became more sympathetic* to Serena and tried to help her find ways to learn.

Serena's parents had consulted numerous mental health professionals, but usually in order to support their own positions in the custody and access dispute. They were suspicious of professionals and also *limited Serena's access to peers and community activities,* for fear that their family situation would become public. They brought Serena to several therapists, but as soon as she began to resist going to appointments or the therapist tried to explore family issues, *therapy would be terminated.* Since the recent violent incident, however, they indicated they would try harder to work together for their daughter's benefit. Serena herself was *superficially cooperative* with interviews but generally mistrusted therapists, along with other adults.

In response to the consultation question "query bipolar child" I answered "unlikely." I reviewed the diagnoses but also provided a case formulation. I described Serena's difficulties as due to a *chronic inability to regulate emotions* (anger, anxiety, and sadness) and attention. Her difficult temperament and language-related learning difficulties were predisposing factors. Most children use *language and executive functions (higher-level cognitive abilities) to regulate feelings and attention, and Serena was delayed in these areas.* A calm, structured environment with predictable, secure attachments further helps children develop affect regulation, and the prolonged and sometimes violent conflict between Serena's parents clearly interfered with such an environment. Serena's early attachment was also compromised by maternal depression. The parents' behavior management strategies were inconsistent, further exacerbating misbehavior. The parents also limited Serena's access to the larger social environment, reducing opportunities to develop other secure relationships or see role models of effective coping.

Given these risk factors, Serena was poorly equipped to learn at school. *School failure undermined her self-esteem,* resulting in learned helplessness (the tendency to give up on work without trying) and causing her to gravitate toward antisocial peers. Serena's *mistrust of authority figures* further impacted academic success and also interfered with engaging in therapeutic relationships. *Acting out was also becoming a preferred coping style,* and she showed little motivation to develop better self-control. Serena's popularity among peers and sympathetic teachers and recent parental cooperation on her behalf, however, offered a glimmer of hope. A treatment plan that built on these strengths was proposed.

CHAPTER 5

Social Aspects
of the Formulation

Social aspects of the formulation pertain to human relationships that impact the child's development. Relationships are considered broadly to include those within the child's family, between the child and school personnel or day care providers, between the child and his peers, and between the child and family and the local community or people in general. As mental health providers, we form relationships with our clients and their families, so we too have a role to play in the child's social environment. In this chapter, each of these social influences is considered in turn, and some possible interactions among them are illustrated using a case example.

FAMILY INFLUENCES

In Chapter 4, aspects of parenting that affect children's development were discussed, and the role of the family in development was introduced. In particular, the family's role in regulating the relationship between the child and all other social influences was highlighted in Figure 4.1. Children's experiences within the family itself can, however, also have profound effects on their development. Therefore, experiences and interactions within the family are now examined in more detail.

Circularity

Although there are numerous theories about what constitutes family health and family dysfunction, most agree that family interactions are often circular. That is, family members react to one another and elicit reactions from one another in ways that make it difficult if not impossible to determine who started the interaction. For example, a young teen may spend a great deal of time alone in her room and her father may worry about what she is doing in there. The father asks increasingly specific questions about his daughter's activities. The girl, who is in the process of developing greater autonomy from her family, finds the questions intrusive and so answers evasively. The evasive answers fuel her father's worries about her activities, prompting more questions and, in turn, more evasive responses. The more he pursues answers, the more the girl withdraws. Similar pursuit–withdrawal patterns can occur in families of younger children around doing homework and completing other daily tasks. The more the parents remind and nag the child about doing the task, the more the child tries to avoid the work. Other common circular, self-perpetuating patterns include excessive parental reassurance that undermines child confidence and results in clingy child behavior, which then prompts more parental reassurance; or parental withdrawal resulting in attention-seeking behavior by the child, prompting further parental withdrawal; or parental criticism undermining child self-esteem and ability to succeed, prompting further parental criticism.

All of these patterns can also be described as starting with the child's behavior rather than the parent's behavior. It doesn't matter. By the time the family reaches your office, asking who started the pattern is as futile as asking whether the chicken or the egg came first. Therefore, it is important to identify the pattern and explain it to the family without assigning blame.

These circular interactions are not limited to parent–child interactions. They can also occur between spouses and among siblings and other family members. In addition, dyadic patterns of interaction can draw in other family members, resulting in more complex patterns. For example, a sibling conflict will often pull in parents as they intervene to avoid harm to one or both children. A parental conflict sometimes contributes to emotional symptoms in a child who may then (usually without conscious awareness) magnify the symptoms to distract the parents from their conflict. This latter pattern has prompted many mental health clinicians to routinely ask themselves the question "Do the child's symptoms serve a purpose in the family context?" as part of a thoughtful assessment.

Closeness and Distance in Family Relationships

It is important to note that circular interactions are not always conflicted. Sometimes, a circular interaction serves to reinforce patterns of closeness and dependency among family members. For example, children who avoid going to school because of separation anxiety sometimes report having an ill or disabled parent at home. Predictably, the parent's condition deteriorates whenever the child begins attending school consistently, resulting in increased separation anxiety in the child, further school avoidance, and increasing mutual dependency between parent and child. Lack of awareness of this type of interaction can result in repeated futile attempts to return the child to school and increasing frustration among mental health professionals and school personnel.

A further detrimental aspect of overly close dyadic relationships is their potential to make other relationships in the family more distant. For example, as a child becomes overly focused on one parent, her relationship with the other parent may deteriorate. Thus, there is no longer an opportunity for one parent's weaknesses to be offset by the other parent's strengths, and the child's development becomes unduly influenced by the characteristics of the closer parent. The marital relationship may also deteriorate in this scenario, as the more distant parent feels neglected by his or her partner.

Families and Psychopathology

Children's mental health symptoms can generally increase or decrease in response to family dynamics, but certain aspects of family functioning have been associated consistently with certain types of child psychopathology. Some reported regularly include:

- Overprotective or overly controlling parenting associated with childhood anxiety disorders (Hudson & Rapee, 2001).
- Parental rejection or lack of warmth associated with childhood depression (Magaro & Weisz, 2006).
- Neglectful/punishing parenting associated with child delinquency (Hoeve et al., 2008).

The above associations, however, do not always imply causality. Although it is possible that certain family styles contribute to children's mental health problems, it is also possible that families may appear dysfunctional in response to children's difficulties or the treatment of those difficulties. For example, families of children who are hospitalized for severe emotional disturbances often appear conflicted and dysfunctional in the context of the child's hospitalization (a highly stressful event for any family). When seen several months later after the child's condition has improved, the same families may appear emotionally healthy and helpful to their children.

Family styles may also be influenced by parents' own psychological problems and psychiatric disorders and so may not be entirely within the parents' control. For example, parents who struggle with substance abuse or anxiety disorders often have children prone to the same disorders due, at least in part, to their modeling of behaviors linked to those disorders (Chassin, Rogosch, & Barrera, 1991; Rapee & Melville, 1997). Similarly, parents with insecure attachment histories may have difficulty developing relationships with their children that are warm, secure, and not overprotective. This difficulty may place their children at risk for internalizing disorders (Hudson & Rapee, 2001; Magaro & Weisz, 2006).

Parenting that is considered optimal may also vary from one culture to another. For example, parenting considered overly authoritarian by North American standards may be considered normative in some cultures. There, a loving parent would not see the imposition of strict rules as being harmful to his or her child and might perceive a more laissez-faire parenting style as neglectful. Family immigration to North America, however, could result in a clash between local childrearing expectations and those of the culture of origin.

Protective Family Characteristics

Certain family characteristics are almost universally helpful in aiding children's healthy psychological development. These characteristics represent family-based protective factors in case formulation. Common ones include:

- Secure parent–child attachments.
- Stable and supportive marital relationships.
- Consistent family rules and routines.

- Clear and respectful communication among family members.
- Clear roles and responsibilities for family members.
- Comfort with emotions: the ability of family members to express and deal with feelings.
- Emotional warmth.
- Successful methods for solving family conflicts and other family problems.
- Some tolerance for variation in individual family members' characteristics and preferences.
- Flexibility in dealing with change, including change related to children's development.
- Connection with supportive friends and/or a supportive community (sometimes also includes supportive extended family members).
- Enjoyment of some regular time together as a family (e.g., family dinners, weekend outings).

Nevertheless, we must recognize that lack of time, money, or parental energy can strain the coping abilities of even high-functioning families. Therefore, it is important to inquire about these resources when examining families' ability to support their children's emotional development.

SCHOOL AND DAY CARE INFLUENCES

School-age children spend much of their waking life at school, and preschoolers spend a substantial amount of time with day care providers. Next to the family, schools and day care centers therefore have the greatest potential to influence children's development.

School-Related Mental Health Challenges

School-related mental health problems constitute a large proportion of clinical practice with children. Some disorders, such as ADHD and learning disabilities, manifest regularly in school settings. Many others, however, can affect school performance. For example, longitudinal studies show that children with anxiety disorders are at increased risk of academic failure (Ialongo, Edelsohn, Werthamer-Larsson, Crockett, & Kellam, 1995), and declining academic performance is a common symptom of teen depression. In fact, mental health difficulties are one of the strongest predictors of academic failure and school absenteeism in youth (DeSocio & Hootman, 2004). Moreover, clinicians often underestimate the developmental challenges posed to children at school entry. The ability to separate from the home environment without distress, to remain seated and attend to an adult for long periods of time, to successfully interact and work cooperatively with diverse peers, to navigate around a large school building, to eat outside the home and in front of others, and to know and follow the rules of common athletic games are just a few of these challenges. Small wonder that many common mental health problems first come to clinical attention shortly after children start school!

Protective Influences at School

The school environment can enhance or detract from children's achievement and mental well-being. A recent summary of meta-analyses in this field suggests that teachers are the most influential element in this process (Hattie, 2009). Teachers cannot take the place of counselors or therapists, but they are often excellent observers of children's symptoms and progress and can sometimes participate in behavioral interventions in collaboration with mental health professionals (e.g., by positively reinforcing desired behavior). The most helpful teachers have been found to provide regular constructive evaluations of what is or is not effective for students, cultivate relationships of mutual respect with students, and use metacognitive strategies (i.e., think about thinking or learning patterns to solve problems; Hattie, 2009). They also avoid labeling students and engage in ongoing professional development of their teaching skills.

In some cases, an excellent teacher also serves as a role model or mentor for the child, potentially buffering the effects of an unhappy home life. For example, a child from a critical or rejecting family environment may have a teacher who notices and nurtures a special talent that child possesses. Developing that talent increases the child's confidence and self-esteem, serving as a protective factor that may reduce the child's risk of depression. Without family support, however, the benefits may not last beyond the child's time at that teacher's school, or the child may become overly dependent on praise related to the talent (i.e., feel worthy only when performing well). A great school environment can usually not compensate completely for an unhappy one at home.

Other school influences conducive to student achievement and well-being include having clear, structured classroom management and routines, allowing students to work with peers of the same mental age, smaller school size, mainstreaming of special education students, encouraging students' understanding of their own achievement, fostering students' abstract reasoning, and strategies to build students' academic motivation (Hattie, 2009). Plenty of advance notice for tests and assignments generally reduces anxiety, which is also helpful to most students.

School-Related Risks

Some school settings can be distressing for children. Schools that foster excessive competition among children (either academic or athletic), that fail to address bullying, or that fail to tailor teaching to the child's learning needs can all harm rather than nurture children's healthy emotional development. For example, schools that limit accommodations for students with learning disabilities because they do not want to provide them an "unfair advantage" are both fostering unhealthy competition among students and showing a clear disregard for their learning needs. Rigid school policies concerning classroom attendance can be disadvantageous to students struggling with severe mood or anxiety disorders, who may need to gradually progress from partial to full attendance or from working in an office or library setting to working in the classroom. Successful interventions to address bullying almost always require a systemic, schoolwide approach (Englander, 2012). When schools merely punish offending youth, the bullying often continues, although in a more covert manner.

Effective communication between home and school is essential to the care of children with emotional or behavioral problems. Parents may need to be encouraged to advocate on their children's behalf, especially in large or impersonal school settings where teachers can easily lose track of individualized aspects of children's education. In these settings, accommodations agreed upon at parent–school meetings are sometimes not implemented unless parents follow up with the relevant school personnel. Changes in the child's academic performance may also need to be tracked by parents to ensure that any problems are addressed early and that the child's type and level of educational support continues to be appropriate. Mental health professionals can support parents' efforts and provide helpful advice to schools, but few have the time to ensure that the advice is followed consistently.

Transitions from one school environment to another (e.g., from elementary to middle school or middle school to high school) can be particularly challenging for children. Large schools can seem overwhelming for anxious children, and adapting to a rotary system of multiple teachers (vs. working with the same teacher in the same class all day) can be difficult for them as well. Increased responsibility for organizing themselves and working independently can make high school challenging for children with ADHD or learning disabilities. Exposure to an older, more diverse peer group can be daunting for many children as they enter high school.

School-Based Mental Health Interventions

School-based mental health interventions may target these difficult transitions, as well as students with certain mental health risk factors, students with subclinical psychiatric symptoms (called "indicated intervention"), or all students (called "universal intervention"). Evidence suggests that universal programs (e.g., programs teaching relaxation, mindfulness techniques, conflict resolution, empathy, or basic emotion regulation strategies) can help to increase protective factors in students, but indicated and targeted programs are more effective in reducing specific problems (Bagnell & Bostic, 2009). When seeing a child who has participated in a school-based mental health program, it is important to ascertain what exactly was done, who ran the program (and their level of training and supervision), how many of the program skills the child retained or continues to use, and how the program was regarded by students. Sometimes, attending a special program can be perceived as stigmatizing, undermining the potential benefits of the program. Sometimes programs are perceived as normative or even positive. Timing of the program in relation to the academic parts of the day should also be explored. If students miss the same class repeatedly, mental health programs may actually interfere with academic progress. For example, I once saw a young girl who had attended a school-based cognitive-behavioral group for anxiety that consistently coincided with her math class. Ironically, her only remaining anxiety was the fear of failing math! The potential value of structured, well-supervised after-school activity groups should also be considered. In some cases, children participating in such groups show symptomatic improvements comparable to those for mental health programs (Manassis et al., 2010).

PEER INFLUENCES

Families and schools may influence children's development toward what is considered socially normative behavior at the time, but ultimately young people must live in the world of their peers. Therefore, it is adaptive for children to relate effectively to their peers, not only as friends but also as members of the same generational cohort. Friendships and peer acceptance are distinct but related constructs, and both are considered protective factors in case formulation, as they have been associated with improved self-esteem and psychological adjustment (Parker & Asher, 1993).

Friendships

Friendships become increasingly important as children and teens mature and spend more time outside the family home. Friendships have been related to social competence and leadership ability, reduced risks of peer victimization, and improved academic achievement (Newcomb & Bagwell, 1995; Wentzel, Barry, & Caldwell, 2004). Friendships can also serve as a buffer against emotional distress due to academic or family problems. When a practitioner inquires about friendships, however, children should be asked to clearly define what they mean by "friends." Some children assume that only peers who are very close (i.e., in whom they can confide personal information) are friends, while others consider every child in the same class at school their friend. Thus, some children may report large numbers of friends but receive limited social support. Skills that relate to making and keeping friends should also be evaluated, as the presence or absence of such skills can impact emotional development. The nature of online friendships should also be explored to ensure safe use of social media and other online social contact.

Almost all forms of childhood psychopathology can influence the capacity to form and maintain friendships, but they do so in different ways. For example, anxious children are often shy and reluctant to approach peers, children with ADHD may have difficulty maintaining friendships because their impulsive behavior sometimes alienates friends, and children on the autism spectrum may display odd mannerisms (called "stereotypies") or interact in ways considered socially inappropriate (e.g., not taking turns in conversation or perseverating on one conversational topic for long periods of time regardless of listener interest). Therefore, when parents report attempts to teach the child social skills, it is important to ask exactly what skills were taught.

Learning how to start a conversation requires a different skill set than managing one's anger or impulsivity, and developing the capacity for active listening and empathy requires yet another set of skills. Moreover, some of these skills can be acquired without formal social skills training. For example, athletic leagues that emphasize good sportsmanship can improve anger management, martial arts programs can build confidence and opportunities for peer contact in a structured setting, and "social stories" (Reynhout & Carter, 2006) or the "reporter game" (where children are assigned the task of interviewing a peer) can be used in educational settings to develop perspective taking and empathy. If the goal of improving peer relationships can be achieved in a normative peer environment, any stigma related to mental health intervention can often be avoided.

Peer Acceptance

Peer acceptance refers to social status or popularity within a large group and has been associated with increased feelings of belonging and decreased behavior problems in youth (Coie, Terry, Lenox, Lochman, & Hyman, 1995). It is related to friendship in that youth who have more friends are more likely to be accepted by their larger peer group (Parker & Asher, 1993). However, it is also possible for a child with few or no close friends to be accepted as a valued member of his or her peer group. For example, a child may contribute interesting ideas to class discussions, behave in helpful ways toward peers, or tell jokes that lighten everyone's mood without necessarily forming close bonds with one or more members of the group. Peer acceptance related to such positive qualities should also be considered a sign of strength. Parents are often concerned about the harmful effects of "peer pressure" from their child's peer group, particularly if they suspect antisocial tendencies in the group. Although this concern is sometimes legitimate, it is also possible for peer groups to exert prosocial pressure on their members, for example to support environmental or other worthwhile causes. In group therapy, group members can also support one another's efforts to change maladaptive behavior (e.g., avoiding school) and engage in more adaptive behavior.

Families and Peers

Although healthy peer relations can cushion children against some family problems, family adjustment can also impact the child's ability to form healthy relationships with peers. Relationships within the family help children to form their initial mental templates of all human relationships, including those with peers, and so affect the ability to trust and cooperate with peers. Families can also facilitate or restrict access to peers. Parents' willingness to foster healthy relationships between their children and their children's peers is therefore a key family strength. Parents can do this by modeling social contact (e.g., by inviting their own friends to the home), by arranging playdates and other peer activities for young children, and by communicating with their adolescents about the nature of their friendships and peer activities (including setting limits if needed). Conversely, parents who are socially isolated or discouraging of their children's friendships and peer activities may limit an important aspect of their children's development. This can occur when parents have social anxiety or autistic tendencies, when there is family enmeshment (a family structure in which members are overly dependent on one another), or when there is acculturation difficulty (that is, parents are recent immigrants and are suspicious of local children, resulting in discouragement of child friendships).

Bullying

No inquiry about peer relations is complete without asking about bullying. Bullying clearly hurts children's emotional (and sometimes physical) health, and most of it is never seen by or reported to adults. Children may fear reprisals from the bully or the bully's friends if they "tattle" to adults, and they may be ashamed to talk about bullying incidents, as victims often blame themselves. For some children, more than one interview is needed in order for them to broach this sensitive topic. It is also important to recognize that some children both engage in bullying and, at other times, become victims themselves. Gender differences also exist, with bullying among girls tending to be less physical and more covert (e.g., deliberate exclusion of a girl from a group or maligning a girl's reputation) but no less harmful than bullying among boys (Pepler, Jiang, & Craig, 2008). Asking about how bullying is handled by the child's school is helpful, as schoolwide approaches are usually more effective than punishing individual bullies (Pepler et al., 2008).

Cyberbullying can be particularly hurtful and has garnered considerable media attention. Many children and adolescents now access social networking sites and/or communicate through texting. Most of this online communication supports existing friendships and enhances social connectedness among youth (Valkenburg & Peter, 2009). Some youth, however, take advantage of others who use social media by, for example, publicizing private information or images, posting false information, or engaging in intimidation online. Youth can also be vulnerable to predatory adults who may pose as peers online to facilitate meetings with children or adolescents. As in all forms of bullying, however, children must be encouraged to report what has happened to adults. Adults' responses should emphasize ending the bullying (e.g., by "unfriending" the offender online and saving the evidence of bullying in case further action is required) rather than criticizing the victim for making foolish choices online (e.g., by posting personal information that was used by the bully).

THE INFLUENCE OF MENTAL HEALTH PROFESSIONALS

As mental health professionals engaged in case formulation, we usually think of ourselves as observers of the child and family. We rarely acknowledge that we also participate in the predicaments we observe, and our actions can sometimes exacerbate as well as ameliorate children's suffering. Mental health professionals and the systems of care in which they practice are an important part of the child's social environment.

Helpful Professional Characteristics

It has been said that a helpful professional is able, affable, and available (Nelson, 2011). Professional standards usually emphasize the first of these ("ability," or competence in one's professional skills), but to the client the second and third (i.e., affability and availability) may be almost as important. Showing empathy for the plight of the child and his or her family can be challenging, especially in the case of demanding or uncooperative clients, but it is essential to our work. When clients do not feel understood, even the most brilliant case formulation may fall on deaf ears. Availability is crucial in the care of children, as a time delay of even a few months can represent a significant span in a young child's development. For example, 6 months in the life of a 2-year-old represents one quarter of his or her life span and includes a host of developmental changes! For the school-age child or adolescent, availability at times that do not seriously compromise school attendance is also important. Therapists who repeatedly pull children out of the same class at school, for example, can contribute to school failure and thus inadvertently do more harm than good.

Harmful Professional Characteristics

One professional attribute that is often neglected in children's mental health care is the capacity to follow clients over time. Mental health professionals who engage in case formulation, including this author, often enjoy solving puzzles. Indeed, putting together the pieces of a complex formulation is a satisfying intellectual activity. The satisfaction of solving the "puzzle" of a child's presentation, however, must not blind us to the need to provide compassionate care for that child over a number of months and sometimes years. Apart from the mildest conditions, most children's mental health problems require long-term attention and follow-up as the child matures to ensure optimal care for the child and to support the family's ability to cope with the child's illness. Moreover, the care needed for a 6-year-old with a chronic mental health problem is very different from that needed by the same youngster at age 16. Flexibly adapting mental health care to children's development is an important skill that usually requires expertise not only as a therapist but also as a case manager. Without longitudinal follow-up that includes case management, families often "bounce" from one professional to another, resulting in sporadic, uncoordinated mental health care for the child. In addition, important changes in the child's presentation may be missed, assessment procedures may be unnecessarily repeated, and the child and family's trust in mental health providers may be gradually eroded.

Other professional actions that can represent risk factors in children's mental health include:

1. When communicating with children and families:
   - Providing large numbers of suggestions without determining the feasibility of implementing the suggestions or indicating which ones can or cannot be implemented concurrently.
   - Suggesting interventions without determining whether there are resources in the child's local area to provide them (e.g., some evidence-based psychotherapies may not be available in rural or remote areas).
   - Suggesting interventions that require more financial resources than the family can afford.

- Failing to point out the child and family's strengths, resulting in discouragement.
- Providing overwhelming amounts of recent information on the child's condition without sorting the "forest from the trees."
- Assuming that parents know more about the child's condition than they do (which commonly occurs when parents are well educated and/or in the mental health field themselves).
- Implying that the parent is ill informed (e.g., saying "You mean you haven't done X?").

2. When planning treatment:
- Ordering multiple, complex investigations without considering the possible effects of ongoing investigations on child well-being and family life.
- Adherence to rigid rules and procedures that do not benefit the child (e.g., insisting that a child be seen by the next available therapist when a therapist with greater expertise in treating the child's condition will be available shortly).
- Referring the child and family on to another professional in your field when this is not absolutely necessary or when there is a long wait list to see that professional (e.g., referring to an "expert" in the child's condition when you are capable of managing that condition yourself, at least temporarily).
- Focusing excessively on reducing the child's symptoms and failing to consider ways of supporting healthy child and family functioning.
- Failing to communicate with other professionals involved in the child's care, including school personnel.

COMMUNITY AND SOCIETAL INFLUENCES
The Community

Most practitioners would agree that community support is helpful to children with mental health difficulties and their families. Nevertheless, we often focus our assessments on the immediate, nuclear family and assume that supporting the child's progress depends almost entirely on it. Parents, in turn, often assume that they are responsible for raising their children with little or no outside help. However, family friends, neighbors, extended family members, religious organizations, leaders of after-school activity programs, and other community members and groups can all play an important role in supporting children's healthy development and that of their families. Families are often surprised by how willing friends and neighbors are to help, if they only ask. Parents can often exchange support as well, for example, when agreeing to each drive their children to school 1 day a week (i.e., carpooling) or agreeing to take turns babysitting one another's children to allow for some parental respite.

Societal Influences

Societal influences on children's presentations are sometimes considered outside the purview of mental health care. Although it's true that we may not be able to address these influences with evidence-based treatments, it is still important to recognize their impact on children's development and well-being. Moreover, many practitioners feel compelled to advocate on behalf of clients when they suffer needlessly because of societal disadvantages.

Poverty is a pervasive source of disadvantage, impacting children's physical, mental, and emotional health. In fact, rates of mental disorders are higher among children receiving social assistance than in the general population (Spady, Schopflocher, Svenson, & Thompson, 2001). Poverty may also reduce access to necessary treatments for developmental and mental health conditions, as such treatments can be costly and are not always covered by insurance companies or government health plans. Moreover, families living in poverty must often focus their energies on obtaining the necessities of life, making it difficult for them to prioritize child mental health treatment.

Other potential disadvantages that practitioners should keep in mind relate to prejudices children may face. Racism, sexism, homophobia, and negative attitudes toward those with disabilities can all adversely impact children's emotional development. Stigma concerning mental health or developmental problems and their treatment can pose further challenges to children with such problems and their families. Even when prejudice and stigma are not publically condoned, subtle biases may persist. For example, parents of children with problems that cause inconvenience to schools or care providers (e.g., delayed toileting) are sometimes told that their child's developmental needs cannot be met and encouraged to take the child elsewhere without being given a precise reason. Similarly, parents may be told that their child would be more comfortable in a setting with similar peers, resulting in exclusion of disabled or minority children from the mainstream.

Even families that are relatively affluent and do not face social stereotypes can struggle with societal pressures. Finding "family time" for members to enjoy one another's company, for example, or even time for the family to eat a meal together can be challenging in some households. In most two-parent households, both parents work outside the home to support the family, and children shuttle back and forth between home, school, and various child care providers. Single-parent households, in which time pressures and financial pressures often co-occur, can be even more stressful. In addition, children and adolescents may be expected to engage in numerous extracurricular activities in order to obtain acceptance at preferred colleges, resulting in parents spending long hours chauffeuring their youth. In some jurisdictions, youth volunteer work is also (ironically) mandatory for high school graduation. Moreover, many religious institutions, parent–teacher associations, scouting or other youth groups, and other organizations that have traditionally supported family life are in decline, often because people feel they are "too busy" to join them. Questions about family routines and supports are therefore highly relevant to children's mental health.

CASE EXAMPLE: MAX

Some of the interactions that can occur among various social factors in children's lives will now be illustrated with the case of Max, a young boy on the autism spectrum. A vast number of such interactions is possible, so not all can be illustrated, but we hope enough are presented to illustrate the "domino effect" that can occur among adverse social influences as one factor increases the risk of encountering another. Figure 5.1 summarizes the risk and protective factors, and a blank form is provided (Figure 5.2) to facilitate recording social influences in your own cases. Key factors from the table are *italicized* in the story below.

Max was born to a *stressed, dual-career couple* as the second of two *closely spaced children*. Both parents described themselves as *"shy when younger"* and had met at a convention for fans of a popular science fiction television show, but there was no history of diagnosed psychiatric disorders in the family. Max's mother was delighted to have a second son; his father saw the new baby as a source of added stress and cost. Max had an *easy temperament*, though, and was far less demanding than

Factor Type	Risk Factors	Protective Factors	Impact
Biological [Note: all are common among children on the autism spectrum]	• Autistic traits in parents (genetic predisposition), sensory sensitivity, language delay, poor coordination	• Placid, easy temperament as an infant	• Max's parents found him likable, but worried (appropriately) about his progress
Psychological	• Easily overstimulated (by peers, by immersion in water, etc.) so very resistant to changes in the environment	• Secure attachment with both parents	• Avoidance of change or novelty • Limited ability to communicate distress, so becomes increasingly defiant
Family	• Stressful lifestyle, closely spaced children, sibling rivalry	• Intact, educated, motivated to help son • Can work with mental health providers	• Increasingly distant father • Increasingly overburdened mother • Parents persist in efforts to help Max
School/day care	• Little experience with behavioral problems like Max's, so threaten to suspend him	• Notify Children's Aid Society promptly to address suspected abuse	• Mother reacts to day care's actions by seeking mental health assessments for Max • Assesments increase family financial burdens
Peers	• Often behave in overstimulating or unpredictable ways, so Max avoids them	• Don't bother Max or violate his comfort zone	• Most of the time, Max is isolated but content
Mental health professionals	• Lack of follow-up • Many recommendations but not all are feasible • Reluctance to diagnose young child	• Provide speech therapy, occupational therapy, and psychological assessments • Diagnosis provided eventually	• Family becomes increasingly stressed (emotionally and financially) trying to manage a child with unclear but persistent problems • Marital discord and maternal stress prompt abusive incident

Community and society	• Family isolated from community • Long wait lists for publically funded services for Max • High cost of private services for Max	• Supports for child and family available once Max has a diagnosis	• Family stresses (emotional and financial) eventually decrease, and appropriate planning for Max's development occurs

FIGURE 5.1. Risk and protective factors in the formulation for Max, a boy on the autism spectrum.

his brother. He smiled readily and seemed content to observe life from the sidelines.

His parents *saw Max as a "perfect baby"* until he turned 2, when his pediatrician expressed concern that Max was *not yet speaking*. Max's hearing was found to be normal, so a referral was made for a speech–language assessment at the local hospital. Four months later, Max's mother called the hospital to inquire about the referral and was told the family would need to wait 6 more months for the assessment. She asked the pediatrician if the matter could be expedited and was told bluntly, *"Sure, if you write a check."*

She did, and so began a series of developmental assessments by various private practitioners. In addition to his speech delay, Max appeared *poorly coordinated, extremely sensitive* to noise and certain food textures, fearful of slides and other playground equipment, and *reluctant to interact with other children at his day care as they often behaved in unpredictable ways.* Despite intensive *speech therapy and occupational therapy,* he did not say his first words until he turned 3, and his sensory and coordination problems persisted.

The day care provider also alerted Max's parents to the fact that he was having increasingly severe temper tantrums when asked to change from one activity to another. She *threatened to suspend him from the day care* unless the family "got him some help." Once again, *wait lists at the local hospital were long,* so Max's mother arranged for a private psychological assessment, checkbook in hand. The psychologist concluded that Max had a mild general developmental delay, and *recommended more* occupational therapy, a specialized (and rather expensive) day care placement, a parenting course to manage the boy's increasingly difficult behavior, regular play dates with peers to improve socialization, and a program of exercises to stimulate his cognitive development. *No further psychological follow-up was arranged.* When asked about other diagnostic possibilities, the psychologist replied, "Some people

Factor Type	Risk Factors	Protective Factors	Impact
Biological			
Psychological			
Family			
School/day care			
Peers			
Mental health professionals			
Community and society			

FIGURE 5.2. Social aspects of the formulation.

might think that your son could be on the autism spectrum, but he is so friendly and pleasant to work with . . . I think it's unlikely."

Max's parents followed all the recommendations apart from the play dates, as they were quite *isolated from their community* and did not have any friends with children. It was becoming increasingly *difficult for Max's mother to continue working,* however, given the amount of time she was directing to her son's care and development. Max's brother was also developing behavior problems, as he *resented the amount of parental attention his sibling received.* Max's *father became increasingly distant* from the family and increasingly focused on managing the mounting debts.

One day, just after turning 5, Max appeared uncomfortable at day care and pulled his shirt off. He had a large red mark on his back. Max's explanation of the injury was "Mommy made me take a bath." The day care provider *called the Children's Aid Society (CAS)*, suspecting child abuse. The CAS social worker interviewed each family member separately and gathered information from all professionals who had ever seen Max in order to determine whether or not Max needed to be removed from the home. Max's mother immediately confessed that she had struggled to get her son into the bathtub and inadvertently injured him in the process. Max always *fought baths and showers because he was extremely sensitive to having water on his head.* Usually, both parents carried Max to the tub together. However, as the *couple had argued* earlier that day, his mother had not wanted to bother her husband, so she tried to bathe Max on her own. She tearfully implored the worker to believe her and was clearly remorseful. Max's father and brother had no further information to add, and none of the professionals who had seen Max reported any prior evidence of abuse. Eventually, the investigation concluded that the mother had engaged in *"an isolated incident of physical abuse,"* the parents agreed to always work together to bathe their son, and the case was closed. There was *no further social work follow-up.*

At this point, despite her husband's objections, Max's mother decided to arrange for one more psychological assessment to get another opinion on her son's diagnosis. The *new psychologist diagnosed Max as being on the autism spectrum* and agreed to follow his development. Max's mother burst into tears, realizing that despite her best efforts her son could never be returned to a normative developmental path. Max's father fidgeted awkwardly, embarrassed by her public display of emotion. However, *as a result of the autism spectrum diagnosis, Max received regular psychological follow-up,* was eligible for support by an educational assistant when he started school, and the family received a yearly tax credit for Max's developmentally necessary assessments and therapies, *easing its financial burdens.* Once the initial shock of the diagnosis had worn off, Max's *parents were able to work together* with the psychologist to make a plan to optimize their son's development.

CHAPTER 6

Spiritual and Cultural Aspects of the Formulation

This chapter offers a combined focus on cross-cultural issues and spirituality. In many parts of the world, culture and spirituality are intimately linked, and your clients will bring their unique perspectives into the therapy. Their worldview often shapes their understanding of mental health and mental health care. The effects of culturally or spiritually based understandings are often subtle but become starkly evident when clients' understanding of mental illness is culturally rather than medically based. For example, what do you do when parents label their psychotic child "possessed" and insist on consulting an exorcist? Before doing anything, it is usually wise to try to understand the clients' frame of reference. Therefore, we examine some culturally and spiritually determined frames of reference in this chapter as they relate to children's emotional development and mental health care. Several vignettes are included to illustrate key points, but (in contrast to previous chapters) a formulation grid is not, as the effects of culture and spirituality often color the entire presentation rather than representing distinct factors.

It is also worth noting that spirituality provides healthy coping resources for many people and has generally been associated with positive mental health outcomes (Desrosiers, 2012). Mindfulness and other spiritually based practices are also increasingly incorporated in mainstream psychotherapies. Therefore, a section on spiritually based coping is included. Interactions between spiritual and cultural factors and other aspects of case formulation are also reviewed, particularly those that can occur around adolescent development. To begin, however, we examine how to broach the subject of cultural and/or spiritual orientation when talking to children and families.

TALKING ABOUT SPIRITUAL AND CULTURAL MATTERS

Talking about spiritual and cultural matters with clients is uncomfortable for many practitioners. We may fear our likely ignorance of our clients' backgrounds, which can lead to inadvertently stereotyping our clients or overstepping our professional boundaries, as many people consider these matters outside the realm of child mental health. In addition, spiritual and cultural matters are not equally relevant in every case. For example, if client and practitioner have a very similar background and the presenting problem has few spiritual or cultural implications, there may be no need to explore this area in detail. It is still important to be open to such exploration, however, and to let clients know that the subject is not considered "taboo," as it may become relevant during the course of treatment. For example, a child in cognitive-behavioral therapy (CBT) for an anxiety disorder might encounter a sudden, unexpected life event such as the death of a family member. Understanding the meaning of this event in a cultural and spiritual context would be important to determine how (if at all) the therapy should proceed.

There are two common ways of introducing a discussion of cultural or spiritual factors when interviewing children and families. Some practitioners routinely talk to children and families about the fact that biological, psychological, social, and cultural or spiritual factors are all important to understanding the child's difficulties and will therefore all be discussed. Then, when reaching the cultural/spiritual part of the interview, they ask open-ended questions about this area such as "What aspects of your culture or spirituality do you feel connected to?" or "What do you value/not value about the culture you were raised in?" or "What do you find meaningful in your life?" or "What is your spiritual orientation?"

A second way to introduce a discussion of cultural or spiritual factors is to relate them to the presenting problem. In this case, the practitioner would ask one or more of the following questions:

"In your culture or religion, how do you understand . . .
- "These symptoms (Do you see them as part of an illness? Do you think there is another explanation?)"
- "What caused this problem?"
- "What will be helpful for this problem?"
- "My role in helping with this problem?"
- "The child's role (or "your role" if addressing the child) in helping overcome this problem?"
- "The family's role (or "your role" if addressing the parents) in helping with this problem?"
- "The role of your faith/God in helping with this problem? What do you think God would want you to do in this situation?"
- "The role of your community in helping with this problem?"
- "Any aspects of the problem that cannot be solved by mental health intervention? How do you think they could they be solved?"

In addition, to clarify the child and family's goals for treatment, it is often helpful to ask:
- "In your culture, how do people think a child should be functioning at this age?"
- "In your culture, how do people think a family should be functioning with a child of this age?"

Although there are a number of questionnaires regarding cultural and spiritual matters, most authors in this field advocate using open-ended questions to elicit information (Aten, O'Grady, & Worthington, 2012). In addition it is important to recognize that ideas and ideals vary within cultural and spiritual groups, so one should avoid making generalized assumptions. For example, one might assume that all Buddhists have a certain worldview, not realizing that there are many different groups within Buddhism, as within any major world religion. Even within one's own ethnic or cultural group, it is important to elicit information directly from the client rather than making assumptions. He or she may not have been raised in exactly the same place, at exactly the same time, or within exactly the same socioeconomic group as oneself, resulting in a very different perspective.

Also, talking about life experiences related to culture and faith is often more informative and less contentious than talking about specific beliefs. When we listen to clients' stories about their cultural or spiritual experiences, we validate their perspective and gain an understanding of how they came to that perspective. Thus, we nurture the therapeutic relationship and develop a deeper understanding of the clients' worldview. For example, simply finding out that the client is an atheist is far less informative than hearing about the life experiences that discouraged or dissuaded him or her from belief in some form of a "higher power."

The most helpful attitude a practitioner can bring to the table seems to be one of respectful curiosity focused on the child and family's values and experiences. Then those values and experiences can be linked to an understanding of the presenting problem and can often be used to support mental health and coping. For example, some religions have dietary restrictions that may not be difficult to maintain at home but can affect children's socialization. If a child is socially anxious, the need to explain to peers why he or she cannot eat the same foods as they do can exacerbate the anxiety or result in avoidance of certain peer situations altogether. The child may also be anxious about reporting this difficulty to his or her parents, for fear of displeasing them. It is important to interview children separately about cultural and spiritual aspects of their lives, not only in the presence of their parents.

Respectful curiosity also implies a desire to avoid imposing one's own cultural ideas and spiritual beliefs on the client. Occasionally, however, clients will ask their practitioners about these ideas and beliefs. Before answering their questions, it is usually wise to find out why these answers are considered important. Some possible reasons include a fear that the practitioner might not understand the client's worldview (and therefore might not be able to help), a fear of the practitioner trying to sway the client toward his or her worldview, a wish for a common cultural or spiritual bond with the practitioner, or benign curiosity. For some clients, knowing something about the practitioner's life outside the office also represents a way of humanizing the client–practitioner relationship, much in the way that seeing a picture of the practitioner's family in the office can make him or her seem less distant. It is important to be clear about which reasons apply, to address these in a manner that is helpful to the client, and to not provide more information than what the client needs or what one is comfortable disclosing. For clients who persist in their questions, an appropriate response might be "I attend church X and was raised in North America with Y background but have worked with clients from diverse backgrounds and so have some appreciation of the many other perspectives out there. How do you think that fits with your experiences and values?"

As discussions of culture and spirituality proceed, it is also helpful to be aware of the linguistic differences that can contribute to misunderstandings between secular practitioners and religious clients. In other words, the language of cognitions, behaviors, feelings, and coping that is used in secular mental health care sometimes does not map neatly onto related concepts found in spiritual or religious perspectives. Some key differences between these two emphases are shown for the reader's reference in Table 6.1. Further ideas about incorporating an understanding of religion and spirituality in one's practice are detailed in the book *The Psychology of Religion and Spirituality for Clinicians: Using Research in Your Practice* by Aten and colleagues (2012).

CULTURALLY DETERMINED PERSPECTIVES ON MENTAL HEALTH AND ILLNESS

When providing mental health care for children and families from diverse backgrounds, practitioners must recognize that they may not share the same understanding of mental health and illness and the same expectations of treatment as their clients. Depending on the client's culture, mental illness may be interpreted as illness, as character weakness or lack of faith, as demonic possession (as in the example at the beginning of this chapter), as divine punishment, as disability (often eliciting care from the community), or even as a special gift. Definitions of what constitutes mental health or mentally healthy development in a child may vary even more widely. Moreover, the interpretations may differ among members of the same cultural group, particularly if some show a greater degree of acculturation to North American ideas and values than others.

There may also be differences between personal beliefs and the collective beliefs of a cultural group, as people with certain life experiences or personalities may be drawn to certain beliefs. For example, parents who are anxious or have experienced trauma may overemphasize cultural admonitions against allowing adolescents certain freedoms; parents who are hoping for a quick solution for their child's mental health problem may overemphasize their culture's view that the child does not really have an illness. Children's and adolescents' views may or may not parallel those of their parents. Overall, these differences underscore the need to avoid making assumptions. Culturally determined views of mental health and mental illness need to be clarified for each particular child and family seen.

TABLE 6.1. Secular versus Spiritual/Religious Emphasis in Relation to Mental Health Concepts

Secular emphasis	Spiritual/religious emphasis
Mental health	A virtuous life
Thought (adaptive or maladaptive)	Belief (correct or incorrect)
Metacognition (ability to think about thinking)	Appreciation of paradox and the limits of human understanding
Adaptive behavior that reduces distress	Spiritual practice that links one to the sacred (e.g., prayer, meditation, religious rituals)
Personal happiness as a goal	Personal salvation or enlightenment as a goal
Adapting to life's challenges	Accepting one's destiny, accepting the will of God, or doing the will of God despite challenges
Striving to feel optimistic and confident	Cultivating gratitude, forgiveness, and compassion
Self-reliance in solving problems	Collaboration with God and/or religious community in solving problems
Self-worth relates to accomplishment and acceptance by others	Self-worth is inherent in being a child of God (exception: "original sin" doctrine in some forms of Christianity)
Cooperation is important to improve social harmony and make groups more productive	Cooperation is important to bring about social justice for everyone in the human family
Meaning = self-actualization (although it is not always clear what that is)	Meaning is found in trying to live a life aligned with one's spiritual principles
Locus of control (internal)	Doing God's work; being an instrument of peace
Locus of control (external)	Accepting God's will; accepting one's destiny

Expectations of mental health treatment vary across cultures as well (Manassis, 1986). Some cultural views include a bias for or against medication, or for or against psychotherapy. In some cultures, there is a belief that illness should be cured instantaneously or as a result of a single visit. The role of the mental health practitioner differs across cultures. In some cultures, practitioners are expected to be powerful healers who provide answers and cures with little client input. The detailed history taking and collaborative treatment planning common in North

America may seem unusual or disappointing to clients from these cultures. The role of the family in supporting children's progress can be particularly challenging to explain in this context. Cultural interpreters are sometimes needed to avoid misunderstandings, and consultation with clergy or traditional healers from the client's culture may also be helpful.

Even within so-called mainstream North American culture, some people's views about mental health and illness do not fall entirely within the medical model. Many families trust and seek out practitioners of various forms of complementary medicine (e.g., homeopathy, naturopathy, acupuncture), so it is worth inquiring about these alternatives. In many cases, the complementary therapies can serve an adjunctive role to medical or psychological care, although from a medical point of view the benefits may be largely related to placebo effects. Complementary therapies are also typically less symptom focused and more likely to emphasize the child and family's overall well-being, and so don't necessarily compete with traditional care. Some herbal remedies, however, can interact adversely with prescribed medication (e.g., St. John's wort and antidepressants can interact), so it is important to determine exactly what substances the child is being given.

There are certain cultural syndromes that have been described in the mental health literature (American Psychiatric Association, 2013). These syndromes consist of a combination of psychiatric and somatic symptoms that are considered to be a recognizable disease only within a specific culture. They usually have no biochemical basis but do have a specific folk remedy and thus do not always come to the attention of North American practitioners unless the folk remedy is unsuccessful. One example sometimes seen in children or adults of Latin American background is *susto*. This condition occurs in response to a sudden fright (e.g., a fall or accident) that is interpreted as "soul loss." Resulting symptoms include nervousness, despondency, anorexia, insomnia, muscle tics, and diarrhea. There are dozens of culture-bound syndromes like this, so it is less important to learn about all of them than to consider the possibility of such syndromes when children present with atypical psychiatric and somatic symptoms. Then the child and family's understanding of the etiology of the symptoms must be sensitively explored, carefully avoiding the implication that the symptoms are imaginary or the child is "faking" them.

DSM-5 also recognizes a "cultural idiom of distress," which is a nonspecific term or phrase used to talk about suffering among individuals from a certain culture. For example, in some English-speaking countries emotional distress is termed "nerves." In addition "cultural explanations or perceived causes" are culture-specific explanatory models for certain symptoms or illnesses. As with cultural syndromes, it is more important to be sensitive to these possible terms or explanations when they are used by children and families, rather than to memorize a list of them.

SPIRITUALLY BASED COPING

The capacity for communities of faith to provide support and encouragement to their members at stressful times has been mentioned as a protective factor in previous chapters (e.g., in the child with the seizure disorder detailed in Figure 3.3). There are a number of other aspects of spirituality that contribute to coping resources in children and families, however, and some that can interfere with adaptive coping. Before describing these aspects, it must be emphasized that effective work with families who rely heavily on spiritual coping resources usually involves work within their belief system. Challenging beliefs with information or evidence about mental illness is rarely successful, as beliefs (by definition) do not rely on empirical evidence (e.g., a famous Bible verse states, "Now faith is the assurance of things hoped for, the conviction of things not seen" [Heb. 11:1]). There are situations, however, in which certain beliefs seem harmful to the child or family's mental health and may need to be gently questioned (e.g., "I wonder if God is really/always like that" or "How do you know this is what is happening?" or "Could there be another explanation?"). If the client cannot see alternatives within a spiritual framework, gently suggesting a psychological explanation may also be worthwhile (e.g., "I wonder if that is your depression talking" if the client believes in a punitive deity or demon). We now discuss a few examples of such situations.

Pargament, Koenig, and Perez (2000) have summarized key coping strategies that emerge from spiritual or religious worldviews. Most of these strategies buffer against stress, but a few do not. Some that typically buffer include benevolent reappraisal (the stressor has benefits in a spiritual context); collaborative religious coping (problem solving with God); seeking support from God or one's religious community; religious rituals to purify oneself or mark important life transitions; providing spiritual support to others; and using belief to help one forgive oneself or others. Strategies that typically do not buffer against stress include reappraisal of the stressor as punishment from God or as related to malevolent forces; negative attitudes toward God, clergy, or church when stressed; and self-directed rather than collaborative religious coping (e.g., asking God to "fix" the stressor for you when you could do something about it yourself; asking God to take your side in a conflict). Bateson, Schoenrade, and Ventis (1993) have also distinguished as maladaptive the use of faith for self-serving, utilitarian ends (e.g., to gain status in one's religious community), which they term an "extrinsic orientation to faith." By contrast seeing faith as an end in itself ("intrinsic orientation to faith") or as an ongoing quest is seen as more adaptive.

A striking example of benevolent reappraisal in my practice was that of a young man who experienced repeated bouts of chronic illness, became increasingly disabled, and was then mugged by a group of youth, who destroyed his new wheelchair. Although he was angry with the muggers, he did not wallow in self-pity. Instead, he said philosophically, "I've gone through so much and come out OK. God has really blessed me with strength." I had to admire his courage.

Another common example of this strategy is coping with disappointment by telling oneself, "it wasn't meant to be" or "it wasn't in God's plan for me." In situations that are beyond one's control, this means of coping can be very adaptive. Many young children, for example, have limited control over their life circumstances as these are largely managed by adults, and accepting disappointment in this way may be helpful to them. If the situation is one that could be changed, however, this strategy may result in an unnecessarily passive approach. In clients with this attitude, it may be worth asking how they know whether the situation was meant to be or was part of God's plan. As mentioned above, one wouldn't necessarily challenge the client's belief system (in this case, the idea that God makes and monitors individualized life plans for each person), but gently question the absolute nature of the statement.

Perhaps one of the most profound examples of using spiritually-based coping strategies can be seen when children and their families try to deal with the death of a family member. Religious reappraisal may provide reassuring explanations of what has happened. Depending on one's beliefs, explanations could include the belief that the loved one has gone to a better place or is with God or with ancestors, no longer suffering, or moving toward reincarnation, or now belongs to the spiritual substrate of all life. Religious rituals help memorialize the person (e.g., lighting candles, planting a tree, or wearing certain clothing in his or her memory). Remaining family members may feel strengthened by their faith or faith community, which allows them to support one another. The latter is particularly important when parents try to help their children mourn a loss that they may still be grieving themselves. In traumatic grief, where children sometimes suffer guilt about surviving an accident or other sudden event that claims the life of a family member, encouraging spiritually based forgiveness can also help. People sometimes deal with survivor guilt more readily when they recognize that matters of life and death are never entirely within one's control, and that they have already found forgiveness with God or with their spiritual community.

Unfortunately, strategies that serve as poor buffers against stress can also emerge in response to loss, as in the following example.

Case Example: Jorge

Jorge was a 12-year-old boy from a single-parent family, referred for therapy 2 years after the loss of his older brother, Carlos, to kidney disease. He was diagnosed with a mild, chronic depression. When asked about his family, Jorge described his home life as "like living with two ghosts." Jorge's mother, Alicia, had focused most of her energies on managing Carlos's illness, and now that he was gone she maintained a "morbid shrine" to her eldest son, according to Jorge. Alicia did little besides cooking family meals and poring over old photographs of Carlos.

A significant obstacle to coping with the loss was Alicia's insistence that her son's death was part of God's plan. Since it was planned, she saw her emotional suffering as her destiny, so she did not see any point in trying to change it. She also wondered if there was something she had done to deserve this fate. After all, she had prayed repeatedly for her son's recovery and God had still let him die. Perhaps she hadn't prayed hard enough. Perhaps God was punishing her in some way. If so, she deserved her fate, so again, there was no point trying to change it. Discussions with her priest did little to dissuade Alicia from these views. Gently questioning her assumptions about God's plan (i.e., "I wonder if God is really like that," "Could there be another explanation?" and "I wonder if that is your grief talking") only provoked anxiety. She said, "I have to hang on to my faith. I have nothing else to hang on to."

Eventually, as Jorge came to terms with his own grief and his anger toward his mother, and his mother attended a support group for bereaved parents, things began to improve. Alicia gradually found she could "hang on to" her remaining child (Jorge) and a few close friends. She attended church less than before but slowly began to feel better. Jorge and his mother became close once again.

In this case, Alicia's reappraisal of her son's death as punishment from God, negative attitudes about God, and inability to use any helpful spiritual coping strategies kept her stuck in her grief and therefore unable to support her surviving son. Fortunately, Jorge and his mother were both resilient enough to benefit from therapy and other supports, albeit within a secular framework.

Self-directed religious coping (where it is assumed that God or destiny will fix one's problems) is sometimes seen in socially isolated children and families that do not want to risk making changes, fearing failure. In this case, people tell themselves, "I will be rewarded in heaven [or some other version of the hereafter or the future]. Then, God will punish those who are making my life miserable, but I must put up with them for now." The image of God as a judgmental parent and oneself as a favored child can offer some comfort and, to a degree, maintain self-esteem. Unfortunately, it can also reduce one's motivation to make something better of life on earth (given the focus on the hereafter) and isolate people from others. Faith is thus used to justify a limited, emotionally guarded approach to life.

Rather than describing specific strategies, some authors have written about spiritually based coping with reference to ideals that cross religious boundaries (Saint-Laurent, 2011; Armstrong, 2012). For example, most religions contain some version of the Golden Rule ("So whatever you wish that others would do to you, do also to them" [Matt. 7:12]) and encourage empathy and compassion toward others. The inspiration for compassionate behavior varies: one may be inspired by a desire to pay forward the experience of a compassionate God, by the recognition of the sacred in other beings, by a belief in fairness and reciprocity, or by a profound appreciation of the interdependence of all beings that makes it impossible to see another suffer without experiencing some suffering oneself. The behavioral result is the same.

Similarly, most religions contain ideas that encourage believers to relinquish a narrow focus on personal gain and develop a desire to work toward the greater good. This broader, less self-absorbed focus can stem from submitting personal goals to those of God or a spiritual force that manifests in the world through our actions; from feeling worthy in the eyes of God and so lacking a need to prove oneself; from appreciating the sacred in awe-inspiring natural wonders or works of art; from paradox that makes one humbly aware of the limits of human understanding; from perceiving all others as members of the same, interconnected human family; or from mindful attention to the task at hand, moment by moment. Most religions identify intense negative emotions such as anger and fear as obstacles to this broader focus, consistent with recent neurobiological findings that oxytocin (the "empathy hormone" in the brain) competes with the fight-or-flight response in humans (Carter, Lederhendler, & Kirkpatrick, 1999).

Other virtues espoused by most systems of belief include gratitude, forgiveness, hope, and humility. Although religiously inspired virtues do not necessarily always contribute to individual mental health, they often do. Moreover, their practice contributes to our collective well-being, which is vital to supporting children's emotional development.

INTERACTIONS BETWEEN SPIRITUAL/CULTURAL AND BIOLOGICAL FACTORS

Biological risk and protective factors may be interpreted differently by families depending on their ethnic and religious backgrounds. For example, in some cultures medical illnesses or genetic risks are attributed to poor behavior in a past life (called "bad karma") or by the child's parents (the idea of the "sins of the fathers" being visited on the children). Awareness of these attitudes can help practitioners respond sensitively and provide accurate information about disease etiology that may mitigate the emotional impact of such attitudes. Conversely, protective factors such as health, intelligence, and particular talents in the child may be viewed by parents as blessings or gifts to be developed. These parental attitudes can foster children's success but can also result in parent–child conflict if the child is motivated to pursue other goals.

Spiritual and cultural backgrounds can also influence the expression of biologically based mental health problems. For example, the tendency to have obsessions or delusions is based on biological disorders (obsessive–compulsive disorder [OCD] and psychotic disorders, respectively). However, the content of the obsession or delusion may be culturally or religiously determined. For example, an adolescent girl from a strict, traditional Protestant background engaged in compulsive cleaning rituals whenever she heard a particular song on the radio. She eventually disclosed the fact that she knew the singer was a lesbian and reported that obsessive, distressing thoughts about homosexuality entered her mind whenever she heard the song. The distress was clearly linked to her religious background, where homosexuality was considered sinful, and resolved when her OCD was treated. Similarly, a 9-year-old boy compulsively searched the ground for needles whenever he left his home, obsessed with the distressing idea that he would be contaminated by someone else's blood. His parents were members of the Jehovah's Witnesses, who are strictly opposed to blood transfusions. Rather than challenging children's religious beliefs, it is often helpful to put their symptoms into a clinical context by saying something like "That's the nature of OCD. It always seems to pick on things that are totally out of character for you."

INTERACTIONS AMONG SPIRITUAL, CULTURAL, AND PSYCHOLOGICAL FACTORS

Cognitive and emotional aspects of children's development can each interact with spirituality in different ways and are now described, with particular attention to challenges in adolescence.

Cognitive Aspects

Generally, young children tend to have more concrete ideas about faith, often consistent with family background; older children tend to have more abstract ideas that are increasingly independent of family background. Attempts have also been made to describe separate spiritual developmental stages, most notably Fowler's "stages of faith" (Fowler, 1981). Empirical support for separate stages has been limited, however, and the most consistent evidence is for the earliest stages, which show a very clear similarity to Piaget's cognitive stages. Thus, faith is described as "intuitive–projective" in preschoolers, characterized by poorly organized images formed from religious narratives and "mythic–literal" in school-age children, whose religious ideas are organized on the basis of stories and rules that are not critically examined. These descriptions are very consistent with (respectively) preoperational and concrete operational thought.

One consistent observation among practitioners is that adolescents who are capable of abstract, formal operational thought tend to critically examine their own ideas about faith. In part, this tendency relates to healthy striving toward autonomy from the family and development of an independent identity (see below). In part, it relates to the fact that there are so many different, often contradictory ideas about faith that lend themselves to questioning. Inconsistencies are found in all major religious texts, and metaphysics (questions about the nature of the universe and the sacred) has preoccupied scholars for millennia. Many of these thinkers were in their teens when they recorded their most influential ideas (e.g., Descartes's "free will solution" to the problem of why a loving God allows suffering [Descartes, 1641]). Not all adolescents achieve formal operational thought, however, so this kind of spiritual or philosophical inquiry is not universal.

The emphasis on specific beliefs (in addition to practices) in Western monotheistic religions may also provoke more debate in these traditions than in some others. Karen Armstrong (1993), for example, has chronicled historical oscillations between person-like versions of God and more mystical, abstract notions of the sacred in Western thought. The former are conceptually simpler, accessible to larger numbers of people (including those who do not achieve formal operational thought), and often perceived as more comforting but can also be more divisive (as people claim their version of God is best), more prone to being ascribed human failings, and more likely to be seen as controlling world events (resulting in some people absolving themselves of responsibility for the state of their lives and that of the planet). A diversity of concepts may be needed in order for people of all cultures and times to find spiritual solace. By contrast, Eastern traditions tend to emphasize religious practices rather than specific beliefs (e.g., the "Noble Eightfold Path" of Buddhism; Nhat Hanh, 1998). Adolescents striving for autonomy may be more or less amenable to participating in their parents' practices, but debate about specific beliefs tends to be less prominent than in Western traditions.

Mental health practitioners have recently adopted some Eastern practices, with particular emphasis on mindfulness. Mindfulness is a practice that encourages nonjudgmental attention to one's experience in the present moment. Given the contributions of rumination about past events and self-criticism to depression and the contributions of worry about future events and self-consciousness to anxiety, there are clearly potential benefits to mindfulness practice. It is not, however, a panacea. I have seen several adolescents who had been treated using mindfulness techniques alone and continued to struggle because other evidence-based practices had been neglected. For example, anxious adolescents who avoid situations they fear generally continue to be anxious if they do not engage in exposure exercises to face these situations. Continuing mindfulness practices on a regular basis also requires considerable motivation and self-discipline, which not all adolescents (or adults) have.

So where does what we have discussed leave questioning adolescents? Spiritual resolutions vary: some teens return to familiar beliefs and practices, some modify their ideas about spirituality, some adopt alternative beliefs and practices, some move away from spirituality altogether, and others continue to question. Often adolescents eventually come to realize that, just as all parents are flawed, so all systems of belief and practice are flawed, but they may still have value. Faith, by its nature, is fraught with uncertainty. Tolerating uncertainty is necessary, however, if we are to avoid a life of perpetual anxiety, and it is also often a sign of maturity.

Emotional Aspects

Some of the emotional challenges described by Erikson (see Chapter 4) have also been related to faith. For example, God has been described as a trustworthy attachment figure for many people (Kirkpatrick, 1998). Therapists have often observed that clients' gods tend to resemble their parents: people with judgmental parents often believe in judgmental gods and judge themselves harshly; people with close, caring relationships with parents often believe in kinder, gentler gods; and so on. There is accumulating evidence now, however, that belief in God can relate to parent–child attachment in two ways: one's relationship with God may mirror that with one's parents or it may compensate for insecure relationships with one's parents (Kirkpatrick, 1998). In the latter case, people relate to God as a secure attachment figure to compensate for the lack of such a figure when they were growing up, as described in the following example.

Case Example: Perdita

Perdita grew up with a mother who was religious but also quite intrusive, regularly searching her daughter's room and never allowing doors to be closed in the house. She also expected absolute agreement from her children and regularly told her daughter what she was to think about world events, music, religion, and other subjects. If others asked Perdita her opinion, her mother answered for her. Perdita's own personality was suppressed until, in her own words, "It was hard to tell where my mother left off and I began."

Now 17, Perdita talked of struggling with her faith. "I'm so inconsistent. Sometimes I'm completely inspired by God: I'm nicer to people, and even the most ordinary chores seem meaningful. Other times, God is the furthest thing from my mind, and I can't connect with anything. I'm disappointed in myself. I often feel I'm disappointing God too." Her goal was to maintain the "completely inspired" frame of mind constantly, yet she kept sabotaging her attempts to do so by overeating, watching excessive amounts of television, engaging in minor self-injury (superficial skin cutting), keeping an irregular sleep schedule, and generally doing things that undermined her emotional stability.

Eventually, it became clear that she assumed that, like her mother, God wanted to be in control of her thoughts and feelings at all times and would be disappointed with her if she did not acquiesce. Challenging that assumption allowed her to see that, unlike her mother, God could accept her inconsistencies and inability to be "completely inspired" all the time. In her spiritual life (unlike her home life), Perdita could be herself. Ironically, when she gave herself permission to be less consistent, her emotionally destabilizing behaviors decreased, and she behaved more consistently. She also developed a comforting faith in God that offered some refuge from her mother's controlling behaviors.

In Erikson's "initiative versus guilt" challenge, religion is sometimes perceived as exacerbating feelings of guilt, given the many behavioral rules and prohibitions found in some faiths. Yet, the structure provided by a clear, consistent set of rules or morals can be a source of tremendous reassurance for some children. Knowing what is expected of them allows them to feel proud when they can meet those expectations and ask for help or learn from their mistakes when they cannot. For these children, a consistent moral code supports self-esteem and the development of a healthy self-discipline. It is only when the rules are unreasonable or unrealistic for the child's developmental level that they can induce excessive guilt. Developmentally unreasonable expectations might include expecting a preschooler to refrain from reaching for a favorite treat for long periods of time or a bright adolescent to never question or doubt tenets of faith. For example, I have seen several teens who became very anxious about attending religious services when their doubts were labeled as sinful or worthy of punishment rather than being seen as a normal aspect of adolescent development.

"Industry versus inferiority" can be translated, in spiritual terms, as a challenge to work diligently in a manner that is consistent with one's faith or spiritual principles. Although not always defined as success by conventional standards, doing spiritually inspired work can be very satisfying for people of all ages. Children and teens are often surprised at how serving meals at a soup kitchen, tutoring a younger child, or shoveling snow for an elderly person can help them feel good and feel connected with their community. Moreover, people considered unsuccessful or "inferior" in the eyes of society can often find a meaningful place in a community of faith. For example, Jean Vanier has written eloquently about his work with people with mental disabilities in the L'Arche communities (Vanier, 2007). He sees them as remarkable human beings who have much to teach people without disabilities and who can help all of us acknowledge our own vulnerability, brokenness, and need for one another.

Adolescent identity development is a challenge that frequently interacts with cultural/spiritual factors in both healthy and unhealthy ways. Adolescent subcultures focused on anti-social behavior can, unfortunately, attract teens who are struggling with this challenge, as in the following example.

Case Example: Robert

Robert was a bright boy born to an impoverished family in an inner-city environment. He did well at school, but his family could not afford postsecondary education for him. Robert had no clear goals for his life. His father, a manual laborer, criticized him daily and occasionally beat him. He accused him of being a lazy bookworm who didn't know the meaning of an honest day's work. His mother had been sexually abused as a child and had never recovered from this trauma. She cared for Robert but was often unpredictable in her behavior. Robert talked about her with disdain. Robert's parents didn't socialize much. They had few friends and were not close to any particular ethnic or religious organization.

Robert didn't socialize much either, nor did he feel connected to his peer group until he met Colton. Colton was respected and feared in the neighborhood. He led a notorious street gang that violently defended its "turf." Colton took a liking to the intelligent but aimless young man. He showed him his fast car and other luxury items, asked him if he wanted to "make something of himself," and had soon recruited young Robert into his gang. For the first time in his life, Robert felt he had a clear purpose and a sense of belonging. He looked up to Colton, found kindred spirits in the gang, and was able to focus his considerable intelligence on helping his comrades evade police. He knew his lifestyle was risky but preferred his new identity in Colton's gang to his father's disparaging "lazy bookworm" label. He gave up his student identity and focused his energies on the gang.

On reflection, one can see that Robert was an easy target for someone like Colton: a charismatic leader in a violent, antisocial subculture. In a different environment, he could have been similarly targeted by a leader of a religious cult, or of a terrorist cell or other extremist group. Robert's studious temperament did not correspond to the expectations of his working-class parents, he did not seem to have a secure attachment with either parent (in his mother's case because traumatized parents usually cannot form such attachments; in his father's case because abusive parents cannot be trusted by the child), and he was raised in social isolation and poverty with little hope for the future. The gang offered escape from his miserable circumstances, a sense of connection to his peers, and work that (to him) seemed meaningful and suited to his talents. Colton, who seemed almost like a surrogate parent, offered him the hope of gaining the approval and sense of personal worth that his parents were unable or unwilling to provide. In short, gang membership offered a new, ready-made identity.

Spiritual/cultural factors can, however, also contribute in a positive manner to identity formation, as in the following example.

Case Example: Fatima

Fatima was a young Muslim woman who grew up in a predominantly Christian culture. Her hardworking parents had limited time for her but still maintained a warm, close family life. She never doubted she was loved. She was encouraged to quietly fit in with the prevailing culture in order to succeed, but the practices of Islam were maintained at home.

Unfortunately, Fatima was painfully shy and stood out from her peers because she had to wear thick glasses for nearsightedness. She was taunted mercilessly throughout her early school years. She was a very good student but was isolated and felt "like an ugly duckling."

Toward the end of high school, Fatima made a decision: she began wearing the hijab (Muslim headdress). Her parents were initially opposed to the idea, fearing the prejudices of their non-Muslim neighbors. Fatima explained, "I already stand out at school. I'd rather stand out for something I believe in." Her parents understood and eventually supported her decision. Rather than reacting negatively, her peers responded to her new appearance with curiosity. They respected

Fatima for the courage to be unique, a trait often valued by adolescents. Fatima's confidence increased after "going public" with her faith, and Islam became an important part of her emerging identity. However, she did not relinquish other aspects of her identity as she embraced her faith. She continued to have close, supportive relationships with family members, and maintained her academic success and other interests. Her beliefs enhanced her emerging identity, rather than displacing it.

INTERACTIONS AMONG SPIRITUAL, CULTURAL, AND SOCIAL FACTORS

Cultural differences with respect to parenting style and encouragement/discouragement of peer relationships have already been mentioned (Chapter 5), as have culture-specific attitudes about gender preference (Chapter 3) and adolescent autonomy (Chapter 4). Each of these issues can result in family conflict, as children and adolescents from minority backgrounds confront differences between the attitudes of their parents and those of their peers (representing the North American average or majority views). When intense, such family conflicts can harm children's emotional development and sometimes even place them at risk of physical harm (e.g., in some cultures children who are perceived as dishonoring their families are beaten or worse).

Attitudes toward school may also differ across cultures. For example, in many cultures schools are perceived as being solely places of learning, and teachers are respected and even revered. By contrast, North American schools often include athletics, social events, clubs, and other extracurricular activities, and it is common for students to challenge the opinions of their teachers. Pressure for children to excel academically may also be more intense in some immigrant communities than is considered normative by North American standards. In some cultures, expectations of academic achievement are also greater for one gender (usually males) than the other.

Attitudes toward society at large may also be influenced by culture-specific experiences. Refugees from nondemocratic countries, for example, have often experienced maltreatment at the hands of police or other representatives of the state. Therefore, they often regard local law enforcement and other officials with considerable suspicion. In some cases, mental health providers are also regarded with suspicion, particularly when they attempt to communicate with other professionals or agencies on the child's or family's behalf.

Lack of awareness of cultural values can also cause problems for some children and adolescents. For example, I once saw a young teen with no previous history of misbehavior who had been arrested for trespassing. She tearfully explained that she and a friend had confronted a middle-aged woman of Mediterranean descent who was idling her car in her driveway as she talked on the telephone. The teens had told the woman that she was contributing to air pollution and should turn off her engine, as her behavior was harming the environment. The woman angrily accused them of being disrespectful and told them to leave her property immediately. When they did not, she called the police and had them charged with trespassing. The girl couldn't understand why the officer did not uphold the local bylaw that forbade idling, and took the woman's side. I explained to her that respect for elders is a strongly entrenched value in many cultures, and environmental regulations, although very important, are a relatively new development.

There are too many potential examples of different spiritual and cultural factors impacting children's development to detail in one chapter, but perhaps that is not a bad thing. As practitioners, we often do better acknowledging our ignorance and asking our clients about these issues, rather than relying on various sources of information (which are often incomplete) or our own assumptions (which are often incorrect). Asking also gives us a clearer window into our clients' unique experiences, which is helpful for case formulation and is often interesting too.

Finally, you may wonder what I did with the parents who insisted on an exorcism for their psychotic child, mentioned at the beginning of the chapter. After talking to the "exorcist" and determining that the girl would not be abused as part of his ritual, I allowed a short pass for her to leave the hospital to see him. The family understood that medical treatment would continue when their daughter returned to the inpatient unit. By the end of the admission she responded to an antipsychotic medication, I think.

CHAPTER 7

The Process of Case Formulation and Considerations for Preschoolers

This chapter and the two chapters that follow show how to construct a formulation for children at different developmental levels. For simplicity, children are divided by age group into preschoolers, school-age children (approximately ages 6–12 years), and adolescents. In children who are developmentally delayed, however, various factors from a younger chronological age group may be relevant. Conversely, for those who are advanced in one or more aspects of development some factors from an older chronological age group may be relevant. For example, a mature-looking 12-year-old girl may have to deal with attention from older boys, even though such attention is typically an adolescent issue.

Although the focus of this chapter is preschool children, it is also the first chapter in which the process of connecting different risk and protective factors to form a coherent case formulation is discussed in detail. Therefore, it begins with a discussion of this process, then highlights important risk and protective factors in preschoolers (with emphasis on those affecting the parent–child relationship), and concludes with examples of the case formulation process from the preschool age group.

THE PROCESS OF CASE FORMULATION

From the outset, we have talked about the case formulation as a set of hypotheses designed to explain a given child's mental health problems and guide treatment. This book has emphasized the need to systematically collect and synthesize information that is relevant to understanding children's presenting problems when developing case formulations. So far, we have focused mostly on collecting information. Risk and protective factors have been recorded in their respective categories (biological, psychological, social, and spiritual/cultural) with little discussion of how to synthesize them to form a hypothetical model of the child's psychological difficulties. This process of weaving various factors together into a coherent model will now be described.

To start, let's reexamine Figure 1.1 (in Chapter 1), which illustrates the dynamic case formulation. As shown in the figure, the clinician begins by recording biological, psychological, social, and spiritual/cultural risk and protective factors that may be relevant to the child's presentation. These are derived from assessment interviews, questionnaires, and sometimes other investigations, as described in Chapter 2. Given the large amount of information the clinician must organize, using a single table to extract and highlight the most important risk and protective factors is helpful. Often, the blank form shown in Figure 2.1 is sufficient, but sometimes one section of the form is expanded to accommodate multiple risk and protective factors in that area. Thus, if there are many biological risk and protective factors, Figure 3.1 can be used to expand the biological section of the form; if there are many psychological factors, Figure 4.3 can be used to expand that section, and if there are many social factors, Figure 5.2 can be used.

Then the risk and protective factors must be organized into a coherent explanatory model for the child's difficulties. Steps in developing such a model include:

1. Placing risk and protective factors in chronological order.
2. Finding connections among factors, with awareness of which ones are obvious or based on evidence and which ones are more speculative.
3. Writing the case formulation as a story using step 1 and 2 above.
4. Editing the story for objectivity and clarity.
5. Communicating the case formulation and planning intervention based on hypotheses generated by the case formulation (see Chapter 10).

As we have outlined, the clinician proceeds to place risk and protective factors in chronological order with respect to the child's life. For example, if one risk factor is "mother hospitalized for severe depression," it is important to clearly indicate when that event occurred in the child's life. Maternal depression and separation from the family in the child's infancy could severely disrupt the mother–child attachment relationship. Maternal depression and separation from the family in a school-age child would be less likely to affect attachment but could be very frightening to the child and disruptive to the family environment, particularly if the child's other parent was either unavailable or unable to manage the family alone. Of course, maternal depression is also a biological (probably genetic) risk factor for child depression, regardless of its timing in relation to the child's life.

Once all risk and protective factors have been recorded by category (biological, psychological, social, and spiritual/cultural) in relation to the child's life, the clinician looks within and across categories for potential connections among factors. These connections occur when one factor influences the likelihood of experiencing a subsequent factor. For example, within the "social" category, parental separation (a social risk factor) can increase the likelihood of subsequent family financial stress (a second social risk factor). For a cross-category example, consider the effect of a child's constitutionally easy temperament (considered a biological protective factor). Such a temperament style increases the likelihood of positive parent–child relationships (a social protective factor), which in turn increases the likelihood of the child generally assuming others are helpful and kind (a psychological protective factor) and therefore behaving in socially engaging ways, which in turn increases the likelihood of forming friendships (another social protective factor). Protective factors can also ameliorate certain risk factors. For example, spiritual coping through prayer (spiritual/cultural protective factor) may ameliorate anxiety about starting a new school in a child who has a family history of anxiety (biological risk factor) and of being bullied in the past (social risk factor). Of course, in this example the adults in the child's life must also ensure safety from further bullying.

Connections among factors can be clear and obvious or more speculative. For example, when a child with a learning disability (a biological risk factor) encounters a very encouraging teacher (a social protective factor) and subsequently appears happier and more confident at school, it is safe to assume that the teacher's influence has ameliorated some of the adverse effects of the learning disability. By contrast, consider the case of a child who is avoiding school and reports anxiety (a psychological risk factor) and whose parent has recently lost his job and become depressed (a social risk factor) and (during the family interview) appears to feel comforted by the child's presence. One could speculate that the child may feel obligated to remain at home to provide emotional support to that parent, and that this sense of obligation is contributing to school avoidance. This connection is more hypothetical than the first, however, and may need to be revised depending on how the child and family respond to various interventions.

After reviewing all factors and the connections among them, the clinician writes the case formulation as a story. The story begins with the risk and protective factors that occurred earliest in the child's life or even before the child was born and then proceeds forward chronologically. All types of risk and protective factors and all connections among them are considered concurrently. Thus, the clinician does not describe all the biological factors, then all the psychological factors, and so on. Instead, he or she takes a broad view of all factors relevant to the child's psychological well-being at a given point in time, describes those, and then moves on to the next time point.

It helps to put oneself in the child's shoes when writing. For example, a school-age child who is excluded by peers but feels loved and valued within his or her family and community might think "they are just being mean, and I need to focus on nicer people and activities I enjoy." The psychological impact of peer exclusion is relatively modest in this child, as positive family and community relationships are protective. On the other hand, a school-age child who is excluded by peers but has insecure or conflicted family relationships and is isolated from other community members might think "they're probably right. I am a misfit," an interpretation that puts the child at risk for depression.

Finally, the clinician edits the story so that it sounds clear, fair, and objective. In particular, he or she tries to avoid psychological jargon and tries to indicate clearly which connections among various factors are speculative and which ones are based on evidence. Such editing is essential for the clinician to communicate the formulation effectively to the child, the family, and other professionals. Formulations that are unclear or sound biased may inadvertently offend others, sometimes resulting in adverse consequences for the child's mental health care. Communication of the case formulation is discussed further in Chapter 10, including an example of a poorly written formulation.

When editing the story, the clinician also identifies testable hypotheses that result from the formulation. These hypotheses usually relate to the speculative connections within the story. In one example mentioned earlier, an anxious child appeared to be avoiding school because of a sense of obligation to a depressed parent in the home. If this hypothesis is correct, then treating the parent's depression, addressing the family dynamics (perhaps with family therapy), and ensuring daily parental activity outside the home (either seeking a new job or participating in job-related training) should improve the child's school attendance. One would also offer the child evidence-based treatment for anxiety, but this treatment would not be the only intervention provided.

The result of the case formulation process is a coherent story that details the child's psychological suffering and psychological resilience over time and provides one possible explanation of the difficulties and strengths of the child who presents in your office today. This explanation suggests interventions that may be helpful to the child beyond those suggested by the diagnosis. The goal of these additional interventions is to address risk factors that may be contributing to the child's presentation and to strengthen protective factors. For example, children with generalized anxiety disorder usually benefit from CBT, alone or in combination with medication. However, if a child's anxiety is being exacerbated by sleep deprivation, family conflict, and academic failure, then additional interventions to address these factors are indicated. If the child has certain abilities or skills (e.g., being a good swimmer, writer, chess player), then finding a team or club where those skills can be developed may increase the child's self-confidence and thus allow the skills to serve as a protective factor that reduces anxiety. Planning interventions based on the case formulation is discussed further in Chapter 10. The outcomes of these interventions either support or fail to support the hypothetical parts of the case formulation, which may result in revision (a process detailed in Chapter 11).

CASE EXAMPLE: FORMULATING MAX

To illustrate the process of case formulation further, let's reexamine the case of Max, a preschooler on the autism spectrum described in Chapter 5. To begin, Max's risk and protective factors have been ordered chronologically in Figure 7.1 using the simple formulation grid introduced in Chapter 2. Arrows indicate possible connections among factors, and protective factors are indicated with (p).

Let's look at some of the hypothetical connections among factors and some protective elements. These include:

Time	Type of Risk or Protective Factor			
	Biological	Psychological	Social	Spiritual (including cultural)
Remote past	• Autistic traits in parents • Sensory sensitivity • Language delay • Incoordination • Easy infant temperament (p)	• Secure attachment with parents (p) • Easily overstimulated but can't express distress so resists changes in the environment	• Family lifestyle is stressful • Closely spaced children • Sibling rivalry • Intact, educated, psychologically minded family (p)	• Family isolated from community supports
Recent past	• Speech therapy and occupational therapy provided and take effect (p)	• Defiant at day care, especially around transitions • Avoids peers	• Day care threatens suspension for behavior • Peers are overstimulating • Family stress increases • Professionals recommend services but fail to diagnose or follow up	• Long wait lists for developmental services • Parents elect to pay • No financial help without diagnosis
Current	• Autism-specific intervention provided (p)	• Emotional health improves as family stress decreases and there is disorder-specific intervention (p)	• Abusive incident at home • Day care contacts child protective services • Family seeks further assessment	• Financial aid once diagnosis is made (p)

FIGURE 7.1. Formulation grid for Max.

- Sensory sensitivity, language delay, and incoordination that are part of Max's autistic presentation leave him easily overstimulated but unable to express distress, so he responds by resisting changes in the environment (as these could trigger distress from overstimulation).

- Autistic traits in Max's parents result in family isolation from community supports.
- Max's easy temperament, secure attachments, and the fact that he lives in an intact, educated, psychologically minded family are all protective.
- Family stress is increased by the parents' lifestyle, lack of community supports, closely spaced children, and sibling rivalry.
- Max's resistance to environmental change results in defiance at day care, which results in a threat of suspension, prompting his parents to seek developmental services.
- Max's sensitivity to overstimulation results in avoidance of peers.
- Family stress increases as parents elect to pay for private services rather than wait for publically-funded developmental services; professionals also recommend further services but fail to diagnose Max or follow up with the family, resulting in escalating costs.
- Speech therapy and occupational therapy recommended are beneficial.
- High family stress eventually contributes to a physically abusive incident at home, prompting the day care to involve child protective services, which in turn prompts the family to seek a further assessment.
- Max is finally diagnosed as a result of this assessment, resulting in autism-specific intervention, financial aid for the developmental services he needs, and decreased family stress.
- Decreased family stress and disorder-specific intervention improve Max's emotional health.

It is helpful to reflect upon which connections are speculative, both to aid communication with families (where these connections can be phrased tentatively) and to generate testable hypotheses. In this case, for example, the connection between Max's defiance and his sensitivity to stimuli is somewhat speculative. He may be defiant for other reasons (e.g., difference between home and day care expectations, personality clash with someone at the day care), although the fact that defiance occurs mostly at times of transition suggests that environmental stimuli likely play a role. Therefore, when communicating with Max's family we might say, "It seems to be hard for Max to change from one activity to another because change is sometimes overwhelming for him, and that may be why he has been defiant" instead of "Max's sensory sensitivities make him behave defiantly when he is asked to change activities." The testable hypothesis in this case is that Max's defiance relates to his sensory sensitivities. If so, then treating these sensitivities (e.g., with specialized occupational therapy) should improve his behavior. New information about Max or his family could also support or fail to support this hypothesis. For example, if Max's parents consistently give him several warnings about upcoming changes or transitions and Max's day care providers do not, then this difference in behavior management could account for his greater defiance at day care than at home. This new information might result in a revision of the case formulation. It is also possible that both factors (sensory sensitivity and differences in behavior management between home and day care) contribute to Max's defiance at day care. Alternatively, there may be no difference in Max's defiant behavior across environments, but greater tolerance for it at home than at day care. Working with Max and his family over time and observing changes in Max in relation to intervention may be needed in order to test these various hypotheses.

Using the risk factors, protective factors, and the connections between them we hypothesized, it is now possible to write the case formulation as a story. A possible case formulation for Max, already edited for clarity and objectivity, might read as follows:

Despite his constitutionally easy temperament, the sensory sensitivity, language delay, and incoordination that are part of Max's autistic presentation leave him easily overstimulated but unable to express distress. Consequently, Max resists changes in the environment, as these could often trigger his distress. His parents, to whom he is securely attached, are able to sensitively adapt to Max's need for environmental consistency and routine. As they are well educated and psychologically minded, they do their best to provide an environment for Max that minimizes his emotional distress so that he has a better chance of learning and developing his abilities. However, perhaps in relation to parental traits of autism spectrum disorder, they are isolated from their community and so receive little outside support. This lack of support contributes to an already stressful family lifestyle. Parental work schedules, the presence of two closely spaced children, sibling rivalry, and increasing concerns about Max's development are further sources of family stress.

Max is eventually threatened with suspension from day care for defiant behavior. This behavior may relate to his difficulty with changes in the environment or to differences in behavior management between home and day care or both. Max's avoidance of same-age peers (who probably behave in unpredictable and sometimes overstimulating ways) suggests that overstimulation is a contributing factor, although this avoidance may also represent an aspect of his autistic presentation. In any case, facing the loss of a day care space for their son (a further source of family stress), Max's parents urgently seek developmental services. Given the long wait lists for such services in publically funded settings, they elect to pay for private services. However, because their son lacks a formal diagnosis, they cannot receive any financial support toward these costs. Their resulting financial problems are a further source of family stress. However, the speech therapy and occupational therapy services provided appear to benefit Max. Unfortunately, no professional volunteers to manage Max's case long-term, so his parents are left uncertain about how to best meet his developmental needs. All the while, Max's behavior becomes increasingly difficult, and the cost of his care becomes an increasing financial burden, resulting in strained family relationships.

Perhaps due to these strained family relationships, Max's mother attempts to bathe him without her husband's assistance, resulting in injury to Max. Upon noticing the injury, Max's day care provider contacts child protective services. Although the ensuing investigation initially increases family stress, it is also helpful in that it prompts his parents to seek a further developmental assessment for Max, resulting in an accurate diagnosis. This diagnosis prompts autism-specific intervention for Max, financial aid to his family for the developmental services he needs, and eventually decreased family stress. Perhaps because of this decreased family stress and access to disorder-specific intervention, Max's emotional health improves, improving his overall developmental prognosis.

KEY RISK AND PROTECTIVE FACTORS IN PRESCHOOLERS

Having described the process of case formulation generally, we now turn to some specific considerations in preschoolers. It is sometimes assumed that because preschool children have less life experience than older children, case formulation in this age group is simple. In most cases, however, this assumption is false. Risk and protective factors that relate directly to the child may be fewer in this age group, but those relating to the child's environment, particularly the family environment, are often complex. Moreover, because of the crucial role parent–child relationships play in the well-being of preschoolers, obtaining a detailed history of the parents' own life experiences and psychological challenges is also important. To begin, let's review key risk and protective factors in this age group identified in previous chapters. These include:

- Young children show certain temperament styles that are moderately stable but may be gradually modified through interactions with their environment; sudden changes in these styles should alert one to a possible environmental stressor.
- Brain development is rapid in young children and can be affected by genetic abnormalities or genetic vulnerabilities to mental illness, medical illnesses and their treatments, complications of pregnancy or birth, and lifestyle factors that affect development (e.g., adequate nutrition, level of environmental stimulation).
- Young children engage in preoperational thought, which is intuitive and sometimes magical, so they have limited cognitive abilities with respect to concepts of time, planning ahead, and perspective taking.
- Young children's responses to illness may focus on magical wishes or fears about illness; pain and illness seen as punishment, or fear of abandonment by family.
- Young children have a limited number of ways of coping with distress (e.g., act out, withdraw, behave like a younger child, exhibit somatic symptoms) and a limited vocabulary for feelings.
- Young children face emotional challenges related to trust, autonomy, and self-concept and the development of healthy self-control.
- Young children are very dependent on family, especially parents, to navigate these challenges, so mental illness in a parent, unrealistic parental expectations, poverty, or other parental disadvantages, and insecure parent–child attachment can all pose significant risks to children's healthy emotional development.
- As children mature, influences outside the parent–child dyad become increasingly important, including interactions with other family members, preschool or day care providers, peers, and the larger community.
- Cultural expectations regarding the child's behavior, childrearing practices, and mental illness and its treatment are important to explore with families regardless of child age.

- Young children's spiritual concepts are usually concrete and consistent with those of their families.
- Spiritually based coping and support from communities of faith are potential protective factors in children of all ages.

EXPLORING THE PARENTS' PSYCHOLOGICAL BACKGROUND

Given that preschoolers' relationships with their parents are so important to their psychological well-being, the parents' own psychological background is often relevant to case formulation in this age group. The importance of ascertaining a history of mental illness in the parent has already been discussed. Two further aspects of parents' experiences worth exploring are particularly stressful times in the parent's life and past events that might relate to incorrect or exaggerated assumptions about the child. Each of these will now be described.

Stressful times in the parent's life are obviously relevant to parental mental health, but recently they have also been linked to physiological effects on child development. For example, mothers' adverse early life experiences (e.g., being maltreated) can affect the function of the hypothalamus and pituitary gland in the brain, which are part of the body's stress hormone system (Gonzalez, Jenkins, Steiner, & Fleming, 2012). Chronically high stress hormones can change the development of the prefrontal areas of the brain that are responsible for visuospatial reasoning and other cognitive functions important to accurately "reading" infant signals (Hanson et al., 2012). Thus, elevated stress hormones in childhood affect a woman's ability to respond sensitively to her infant when she becomes a mother herself years later. On the other hand, secure attachment in childhood fosters the development of executive functions including those needed to "read" others' emotional signals (Bernier, Carlson, Deschenes, & Matte-Gagne, 2012), thereby increasing the ability to respond sensitively to an infant. Other authors have linked currently elevated stress hormones in mothers with negative, intrusive behavior toward their infants (Mills-Koonce et al., 2009). Being a teenage mother, which is almost universally stressful, has also been linked to suboptimal responsiveness to infant signals (Giardino, Gonzalez, Steiner, & Fleming, 2008). Elevated stress in mothers during pregnancy has been linked to abnormalities in infants' stress regulation and consequent adverse effects on infants' development of cognitive functions that relate to self-regulation (so-called "executive functions"; Egliston, McMahon, & Austin, 2007).

Stressful events in parents' lives do not impact only infants, however. A stable, loving family environment is crucial for healthy emotional development in children of all ages. For example, it is not unusual to see preschoolers develop separation anxiety when their parents are about to separate, or exhibit worsening temper tantrums when there is violence in the home. When parents look after ill relatives, lose their jobs, struggle financially, or are overwhelmed with multiple responsibilities, their parenting abilities are affected. In short, asking about current and past stresses in the parents' lives can be as important as finding out about stressful events that impact the child directly.

Common distorted beliefs and assumptions that parents may harbor about their children are shown in Table 7.1. Such parental biases about the child are important, as they can have adverse effects on children's emotional development. For example, it can be detrimental to a child's self-esteem if the parent assumes the child has flaws that are not really present. Sometimes, this assumption can also be self-fulfilling, as many children eventually behave in a manner that is consistent with parental expectations. Overestimating the child's strengths and abilities can be problematic too, however, as it can leave the child feeling that he or she can never "measure up" to parental expectations. Parents with this bias can also ignore warning signals suggesting serious emotional problems in the child.

Among the most concerning parental assumptions are those that involve severe overidentification with the child. In these parent–child dyads, the psychological boundary between parent and child is blurred, and the child is expected to think, feel, and behave like an extension of the parent. Children in this predicament can become socially isolated, as their lives revolve around their parents, struggle with identity issues (e.g., distinguishing their own ideas and beliefs from those of their parents), and assume age-inappropriate roles as parental confidants. In extreme cases, they may be vulnerable to sexual abuse by parents who no longer distinguish between their own feelings and those of their children.

Other common parental assumptions are that the child is similar to the parent's attachment figure, thus drawing the child into a replay of interpersonal patterns from the parent's past, or that the child resembles a mentally ill relative and will suffer a similar fate. The latter assumption can often be addressed through education about the heritability (or lack of heritability) of various disorders and by pointing out differences between the child and the relative in question. Anxious parents often see their children as more fragile and vulnerable than

TABLE 7.1. Parental Distorted Beliefs about the Child and Their Corresponding Assumptions

Belief	Assumption
"This child is just like me." (mild)	"This child has many of my flaws."
	"This child has many of my strengths."
	"This child's fate will be similar to mine [positive or negative]."
"This child is just like me." (severe; blurring of psychological boundary between parent and child)	"This child has the same tastes and opinions as I do."
	"This child enjoys whatever we do together."
	"This child and I must unite against all who would question our relationship."
	"This child is my best friend and confidant."
"This child is not at all like me." (mild)	"This child has few of my flaws."
	"This child has few of my strengths."
	"This child will have a very different life from mine."
"This child is not at all like me." (severe; parent is unempathic and rejecting of child)	"This child seems strange or alien to me."
	"I cannot understand this child."
	"I cannot trust or enjoy this child."
"This child is just like my attachment figure."	"This child has the same flaws as my attachment figure."
	"This child has the same strengths as my attachment figure."
	"This child is treating me the way my attachment figure treated me."
"This child is just like someone else in my life [present or past]."	"This child has the same flaws as that person."
	"This child has the same strengths as that person."
	"This child is treating me the way that person treated me."
"This child is a source of stress or worry."	"This child is fragile [physically or emotionally]."
	"This child is difficult to parent competently."
	"I cannot give this child what he/she needs."
"This child is burdening me/my family."	"This child is interfering with my school or work plans."
	"This child is adversely affecting my marriage or family."
	"This child is stopping me from looking after my own health or well-being."

they really are, but the same assumption may occur when the child has an actual physical or mental disability or when parents lack support in raising the child. Conversely, children who are born unplanned, who are born at stressful times in the family's life, or who have a difficult temperament can be perceived as a burden by their parents.

Parental assumptions about their children are not always easy to elicit. Some questions to use when starting the inquiry might include:

- "How is this child similar to or different from you at that age? Does this concern you?"
- "Does this child remind you of anyone in your family or anyone in your past?"
- "What worries do you have about this child?"
- "How has having this child affected other aspects of your life?"

Then the clinician can follow up on the responses to further clarify the parents' perspectives on the child's strengths, weaknesses, and possible future, as well as the nature of the parent–child relationship.

Sometimes, however, assumptions only come to light after unsuccessful attempts to educate parents about developmentally appropriate expectations for their children. For example, the idea that a young preschooler is being "deliberately manipulative" toward a parent assumes a cognitive ability to plan and scheme that preschoolers generally do not possess. Preschoolers may habitually engage in attention-seeking or other annoying behaviors, which usually occurs because the behaviors have been unintentionally reinforced, not because of any deliberate plan. Parents who persist in perceiving their preschoolers as plotting against them, despite psychoeducation to dispel this myth, often harbor unfounded assumptions about the child based on their own past experiences.

Such unrealistic assumptions do not necessarily imply a serious mental illness in the parent. We all project our own assumptions onto infants and toddlers to a degree, as they cannot speak up to correct us and we sometimes misread their nonverbal cues. However, the extent to which parental perceptions are based in these assumptions versus the child's actual behavior often provides a clue to unresolved psychological issues in the parent's life. These perceptual issues are worth addressing with parents to reduce the chances of children eventually seeing themselves exactly as their parents portray them, thus limiting their future potential.

CASE EXAMPLE: JASMINE

Jasmine, age 5, was referred for a diagnostic assessment. The consultation request noted "extreme aggression towards family members." A petite girl, Jasmine appeared surprisingly calm and polite at her initial appointment. The "extreme aggression" had consisted of a single incident in which Jasmine was seen brandishing a knife above her baby brother's crib. Her mother had screamed, and Jasmine had dropped the knife and sobbed, "you don't need me any more .. . you only love him!" She was otherwise a well-mannered, developmentally normal preschooler. Her mother noted, however, that Jasmine had been a fussy baby and "No matter what I did, she always cried."

Jasmine's mother and stepfather reported that they had been happily married for 3 years, and both had looked forward to the arrival of the new baby. They reported making an effort to spend time with Jasmine so she would not feel neglected as a result of the baby's arrival. Her mother added, "and I always tell her I love her."

The circumstances of Jasmine's birth, however, had been difficult. Her mother had lived in a war-torn country when Jasmine was conceived. The pregnancy was the unplanned result of an affair between Jasmine's mother and a local government official. He had promised to ensure her family's safe passage out of the country, but did not keep this promise. Several family members were killed, and Jasmine's mother narrowly escaped the same fate. She confessed in private, "Whenever I look at my daughter, I see my sister's face before she died." She still had nightmares about these events.

Jasmine's stepfather was described as "an angel" by his wife. A refugee himself, he had assisted the young mother with documentation and housing, and helped her become connected with their local ethnic community. Jasmine affectionately called him "Daddy" and was unaware that he was not her biological father. After the birth of the baby, Jasmine's stepfather had taken on a second job to support his growing family. He regretted spending less time with the children but felt he had no alternative given the financial pressures on the family. Around the same time, Jasmine started kindergarten, where she was described as friendly but sometimes controlling of other children's games. Since this time, Jasmine had made increasingly resentful comments about her brother.

Figure 7.2 summarizes the risk and protective factors in this case, placed in chronological order with respect to Jasmine's life. The arrows

	Type of Risk or Protective Factor			
Time	Biological	Psychological	Social	Spiritual (including cultural)
Remote past	• Stressful pregnancy • Normal early development (p) • Difficult temperament	• Maternal trauma and probable PTSD • Insecure mother–child attachment	• Stable parental marriage (p) • Stepfather is supportive (p) • Psychologically minded parents (p)	• Parents' successful acculturation after immigrating as refugees (p)
Recent past	• Executive function deficits/ poor emotion regulation	• Feeling neglected • Confused by family secrets • Resentment of sibling • Controlling style with peers	• Birth of sibling • Family financial stress • Kindergarten start • Decreased time with parents	• Potentially supportive community (p) • Cultural openness to mental health services (p)
Current	"	• Aggression toward sibling • Continues to feel confused and neglected	• Little peer support • Family financial stress and little time with parents continues	"

FIGURE 7.2. Formulation grid for Jasmine.

indicate possible connections among risk factors, and protective factors are marked with (p) as follows:

- Difficult temperament, maternal history of trauma, unplanned pregnancy, and probable current posttraumatic stress disorder (PTSD) all adversely affect mother–child relationship, probably resulting in insecure attachment.
- Pregnancy stress may have adversely affected executive functions.
- Difficult temperament may reflect executive function problems or contribute to them.

- Stable parental marriage and successful acculturation have a somewhat protective effect on the mother–child relationship and on Jasmine's well-being.
- Generally normal early development is a positive sign.
- Positive relationship with stepfather has a positive effect on Jasmine's well-being but does not entirely ameliorate the effects of insecure attachment given his absence from her life in the first 2 years.
- Insecure attachment results in difficulty with emotional control and other executive functions and contributes to resentment of sibling later.
- Difficulty controlling her own emotions predisposes her to coping by trying to control the environment, adversely affecting peer relationships, and later contributes to an aggressive response to sibling resentment.
- Family secrets leave Jasmine confused: she is told she is loved but does not feel loved by her mother; she is close to her dad but senses some distance (not knowing he is her stepfather).
- Confusion may result in self-blame (i.e., "If I don't feel loved, I must be unlovable") or mistrust (i.e., people lie about their emotions), further compromising emotion regulation.
- Arrival of brother contributes to financial strain.
- Financial strain results in stepfather taking on a second job, reducing time with Jasmine.
- Stepfather's absence and start of kindergarten make Jasmine more dependent on mother (to whom she is insecurely attached and who is preoccupied with the new baby), resulting in a sense of being emotionally neglected.
- Insecure child who feels emotionally neglected and has poor emotional control blames brother, prompting the knife incident.
- Access to community support and psychologically minded parents are both potential protective factors if developed further.

These connections among factors already provide a point-form description of Jasmine's case formulation. Written in full sentences, it might read as follows:

Jasmine's unplanned birth resulted from very traumatic circumstances in her mother's life that left her with symptoms of posttraumatic stress. These circumstances, in combination with Jasmine's difficult temperament style, adversely affected the mother–child relationship, probably resulting in insecure attachment. Insecure attachment, pregnancy stress, and difficult temperament (perhaps already reflective of problems with self-regulation) all affected Jasmine's development of executive functions, including her ability to regulate strong feelings. Jasmine's positive relationship with her stepfather had an ameliorative effect on her well-being but probably did not completely counteract the effects of insecure attachment, given his absence from the first 2 years of her life. Nevertheless, the stable marriage of Jasmine's parents and their successful acculturation was moderately protective of the mother–child relationship and of Jasmine's well-being. Jasmine's generally normal early development is also a positive prognostic sign.

Jasmine's insecure early attachment and executive function deficits became increasingly problematic as her family coped with the stresses of a new baby and attendant financial problems, all this occurring at a time when there was a developmental expectation that Jasmine spend more time away from home (i.e., attend kindergarten). Financial strain resulted in her stepfather taking on a second job, reducing his time with Jasmine. Her stepfather's absence and starting kindergarten made Jasmine more dependent on her mother, resulting in her feeling emotionally neglected at home. At school, she found little support among her peers. Her difficulty controlling her emotions predisposed Jasmine to coping by trying to control the environment, which did nothing to help her make friends.

Jasmine's insecurities and self-regulation difficulties may have been further exacerbated by confusion related to her family's secrets. For example, although Jasmine's mother tells her she is loved, she may not feel loved given the insecure nature of the mother–child relationship. She may also sense some distance from her "daddy," not knowing he is her stepfather. Confusion might also result in self-blame (i.e., "If I don't feel loved, I must be unlovable") or mistrust (i.e., people lie about their emotions), further compromising Jasmine's emotion regulation.

Eventually, Jasmine blamed her feelings of emotional neglect and confusion on the most obvious target in her life: her baby brother. Insecure attachment to her mother and a perceived lack of emotional support contributed to this sibling resentment. Without the capacity for emotional control, Jasmine lashed out at the object of her resentment, threatening her infant brother with a knife.

In this case formulation, I have tried to phrase speculative connections tentatively, to aid both communication and the generation of hypotheses. If I had not done so, editing would be indicated. The paragraph about family secrets is probably the most speculative, and so the qualifier "may" is used in the first sentence. Moreover, I would not tell

Jasmine's parents to disclose these secrets to her unless and until they were comfortable doing so. Although the truth about Jasmine's parentage is likely to emerge eventually, the pros and cons of sharing such information at different developmental stages would need to be carefully assessed.

With respect to Jasmine's treatment, the above formulation suggests the following:

- Need to treat mother's probable PTSD and traumatic grief.
- Psychological intervention focusing on mother and child (e.g., child–parent psychotherapy [Lieberman & Van Horn, 2008]).
- Need to develop potential protective factors, including psycho-education of psychologically minded parents regarding Jasmine's difficulties so they can support her better, and accessing of community support (e.g., relief from some household chores for mother; occasional babysitting of infant brother to allow time for mother and daughter to participate in treatment and spend time together).
- Positive peer experiences for Jasmine in which she is not in a competitive or controlling role (e.g., Sparks—the preschool equivalent of Girl Guides).

Interestingly, based on this formulation, treating Jasmine's aggression either medically or behaviorally should not be the main focus of intervention. Instead, improved parent–child relationships are seen as the main means of improving Jasmine's well-being. It is obviously still important to ensure the baby's safety, but the interventions suggested by the formulation will result in maintaining safety without subjecting Jasmine to unhelpful treatments. As always, if more factors come to light over time or if intervention is not successful, this formulation may need to be revised.

CHAPTER 8

Case Formulation for School-Age Children

Case formulation for children in the early school years (about ages 6–12) requires an understanding of the many challenges children face as they begin to spend most of their days in educational settings, away from the home environment. These challenges are outlined below, along with a review of highlights from previous chapters pertaining to this age group. Several case examples are included, and clinicians are encouraged to formulate these examples themselves using the steps outlined in Chapter 7 before reading my proposed case formulations.

SCHOOL-RELATED CHALLENGES

As shown in Table 8.1, children require many abilities and supports to function successfully at school. The challenges listed in the table can interfere with school success for most children and thus adversely impact their mental health. Additional school-related challenges can arise in relation to specific psychological problems. Two common psychological problems that can affect school success are ADHD and anxiety disorders. Common challenges related to ADHD include distractibility that impairs work completion or results in "clowning" in class, inability to stay seated, low frustration tolerance, impatience, inability to organize a desk or locker, forgetting homework assignments, talking

TABLE 8.1. Common School-Related Challenges

Environmental domain

- Family values child's education
- Consistent sleep routines
- Organized early-morning routines, including breakfast
- Timely and comfortable transportation to and from school
- Successfully navigating the school building
- Comfortable and orderly classroom

Interpersonal domain

- Ability to separate from home/parents
- Ability to relate positively to teacher(s)
- Establishing and maintaining healthy peer relationships (friends, popularity, freedom from bullying/fighting/exclusion)
- Ability to work successfully in groups
- Ability to integrate with school community/expectations
- Consistent home and school communication/expectations

Learning domain

- Ability to comprehend material and instructions
- Freedom from physical distractions (e.g., hunger, illness)
- Freedom from mental distractions (e.g., intrusive thoughts/worries)
- Optimal level of emotional arousal (i.e., neither bored nor nervous)
- Ability to regulate attention and emotions to allow focused academic work
- Ability to maintain motivation and optimism about academic work
- Ability to work independently but ask for assistance when needed
- Ability to manage presentations and other performance situations
- Ability to organize and execute projects and other large assignments
- Ability to complete assigned homework

out of turn or blurting out answers, and impulsivity that can injure the child or peers. Common challenges related to anxiety can include perfectionism, being overwhelmed by large assignments, test anxiety, anxiety about time pressure, intolerance of uncertainty or events that are out of the ordinary (e.g., field trips, substitute teachers), excessive reassurance seeking, anxiety-related physical symptoms (headaches, stomachaches, panic feelings), and high interpersonal sensitivity. These are detailed further in Manassis (2012). In addition, learning disabilities almost always affect school success and should be suspected in children who present with psychological symptoms that occur mainly in relation to schoolwork.

Clinicians working with school-age children should inquire about challenges in three broad areas: school and home environment, interpersonal situations at school, and learning difficulties. Although these problems may seem obvious, they are easy to overlook, so all of them are described in detail in the order listed in the table.

In a family that values the child's education, a successful school day begins at home. Children who are not encouraged in their studies or not provided with a quiet place to study, or who are forced to look after younger siblings or work in family businesses are academically disadvantaged. Lack of sleep is a common source of school issues including compromised learning, irritability, and lack of concentration. Inconsistent bedtime routines, daytime napping, lack of exercise, use of television or other electronic devices into the late evening, and the consumption of caffeinated beverages (e.g., energy drinks) are common culprits at all ages. Adolescents often present with sleep cycle disturbances, including not falling asleep until the early morning hours, but since the advent of video games and other electronic distractions younger children may present with this problem as well. Children who skip breakfast are prone to learning difficulties, especially in the mornings, so it is worth inquiring about this meal. Morning routines that are chaotic or differ from one household to another (in separated or divorced families) can be anxiety provoking and result in forgetting homework or other school materials or result in lateness. Some schools take a very punitive approach to tardiness, resulting in embarrassment to the child. The trip from home to school exposes the child to another potentially problematic environment: the vehicle used for transportation and its occupants. Children who report disliking school are sometimes reacting to being taunted on the school bus or in the carpool, so it is worth inquiring about these settings. In the early school years, children often attend a single class that is easy to locate. The need to rotate from class to class and to keep one's possessions in a locker with a unique combination is a new challenge in middle school. Children who have limited memory or visuospatial ability may find this particularly difficult, especially at the beginning of the year. Finally, a classroom environment that is physically uncomfortable (e.g., too hot, too cold, too noisy) or where children's behavior is not well controlled can make learning difficult. For example, children who are very sensitive to noise sometimes benefit from having tennis balls attached to the bottom of chair and desk legs to muffle sounds when furniture is moved across the floor.

Children at school must relate to teachers, peers, and groups, but first they must successfully separate from their home and parents. Difficulties usually occur when both parent and child fear the separation, often because the parent lacks confidence in the child's ability to cope.

Experienced day care providers often minimize the problem by limiting parent–child interactions at drop-off time, but children and parents who have not had this experience and are anxious may struggle initially when the children start school. In order to relate well to teachers, children must be polite, participate appropriately in class, avoid engaging in disruptive behavior, know how to ask for help appropriately, and adapt to the teacher's personality and teaching style. Moreover, the ideal teacher for one child may be problematic for another. For example, an inattentive child may become more engaged in a lesson when asked to demonstrate his or her understanding of a topic, but an anxious, self-conscious child might feel overwhelmed by being "put on the spot" in this way. Friendships with peers are important at all ages, as they increase children's sense of social acceptance and esteem, foster the development of social skills, and can also protect them from bullying or peer exclusion. Making friends is often challenging for shy children, but keeping friends tends to be more difficult for those prone to impulsivity or controlling behavior. Some children have few close friends but are still well liked among their peers and seem content with their level of social contact, so if children lack friends it is worth clarifying whether or not they find this distressing.

Working collaboratively in groups requires different skills than managing individual relationships, and is not easy for many children. Making sure everyone's ideas are heard, making decisions as a group, and ensuring that group members do their share are just some of the challenges. Group evaluations add further concerns, as many strong students fear being evaluated negatively when their work is combined with that of weaker students in the group.

Beyond the classroom, children often participate in a variety of extracurricular school activities, which can mitigate or magnify interpersonal challenges, depending on how they are led. An excellent coach, for example, can offset negative experiences with a teacher, but a poorly supervised activity can exacerbate bullying among peers. The values of the school community, often reinforced by the principal, can also have an important impact on children. Good principals can foster a respectful, supportive school environment where teachers and students alike feel valued and motivated. Finally, parents' and teachers' expectations of each other can pose challenges for children. For example, if teachers and parents blame each other for a child's problem, the child does not learn to take responsibility for working on the problem. Conversely, if teachers and parents have realistic expectations of each other and communicate regularly and respectfully about the child's difficulties, the child receives clear, consistent messages about what he or she must do to improve. In practice, given the number of students taught by each teacher, it is usually up to parents to ensure that communication between home and school occurs regularly so that problems arising can be addressed promptly and effectively.

Effective learning requires more than cognitive abilities alone. Comprehending the material taught and teacher instructions is just the beginning of the learning process. Children who are physically ill, hungry, or distracted by worries or intrusive thoughts (e.g., in children who have traumatic memories or have obsessive–compulsive disorder) all struggle to attend to their academic work. Attention is further affected by the child's level of physiological arousal. Children who are either bored (i.e., underaroused) or nervous (i.e., overaroused) do not perform at their best on cognitive tasks. Developmentally, children's abilities to regulate attention and emotion (also called "executive functions") generally improve with age, but some children lag behind in one or more of these areas. Children who are either depressed or discouraged from repeated school failure (also called "learned helplessness," in the case of children with learning disabilities) may lack the motivation, energy, and optimism to persevere with school assignments, particularly when these are large. They often need repeated opportunities to complete small tasks with consistent encouragement in order to restore their faith in their own academic abilities. Most teachers value students' ability to work independently, so intelligent children who lack confidence or seem overly dependent on adults are sometimes evaluated poorly. By contrast, however, students who avoid asking for help entirely can remain confused for long periods of time, which interferes with their learning. Thus, asking for help when needed is a simple but important skill. Presentations, tests, and other performance situations are anxiety provoking for most children, but successful learners are able to tolerate this anxiety and manage these situations. As mentioned, large assignments are particularly challenging for children who lack optimism or motivation, but they can also be difficult for children who lack the ability to break assignments into chunks and schedule work periods for completing them, and lack other organizational skills. As students progress through school, they are increasingly expected to complete some work at home and to review previous work in preparation for tests and examinations. Remembering to bring home required books and materials, having a consistent time and place for homework, remembering to bring the homework back to school, and avoiding family arguments around homework completion are all potential challenges. When family arguments around this issue are severe, it is sometimes recommended that children be allowed to experience the natural consequences of failing to complete the work (i.e., teacher criticism or other penalty). In addition, it may be helpful to involve a tutor who is not part of the family.

Despite its attendant challenges, school can be a wonderful experience for some children with psychological difficulties, particularly for children raised in difficult family circumstances. Here, school represents an opportunity to see a different world view from that espoused by parents. Peers can provide yet another perspective on life, as can the parents of peers. Children are afforded the opportunity to see how other families live and can gain a vision of the different strengths and weaknesses within different families. Moreover, teachers or coaches can serve as role models of caring, competent adults and can help build self-esteem by fostering the child's strengths. School also represents a community with values and expectations that may differ from those of the family. For example, children who have never been given a chore or other responsibility in their families may find that at school they are expected to make a contribution. Being a classroom helper or being a "reading buddy" to a younger child can help children recognize their ability to give to others, rather than always being the recipients of care. In summary, school experiences cannot erase the scars left by difficult home environments, but they can provide alternative experiences that show children that different life paths may be possible.

A SCHOOL-FOCUSED EXAMPLE: REVISITING MALCOLM

At the beginning of this book, the example of Malcolm was presented. As you may remember, Malcolm suffered from ADHD and a possible anxiety disorder. These psychological problems severely affected his school performance, but his difficulties were magnified by family problems and by misguided efforts to provide group CBT for his anxiety. At this point, you may wish to review this example in Chapter 1 and develop a formulation of biological, psychological, social, and spiritual/cultural factors relevant to Malcolm's difficulties and strengths. Use arrows to indicate possible connections among factors and then write the formulation as a story in the manner illustrated in Chapter 7. A sample formulation grid for Malcolm is provided in Figure 8.1. Here is one possible formulation of Malcolm's problems:

Malcolm was born a healthy boy who met his developmental milestones without difficulty. In his early school years, however, Malcolm showed symptoms of inattention that were prominent enough to cause his teacher to suggest a psychological assessment. Noting her son's school-related stomachaches (that are sometimes a sign of anxiety) and wanting to avoid medication (the most common and effective treatment

| Time | Type of Risk or Protective Factor | | | |
	Biological	Psychological	Social	Spiritual (including cultural)
Remote past	• ADHD • Possible anxiety disorder • Healthy and developmentally normal (p)	• Mixed messages from adults, so little motivation to improve his work	• Teacher concern (p) • Parent blaming teacher • Parental conflict and inconsistent behavior management	• Cultural bias toward evidence-based treatment with little regard for context and against psychiatric medication
Recent past	• ADHD • Anxiety disorder	• Heightened anxiety as parents separate • Learned helplessness from ongoing school failure and recent therapy failure	• Negative parental attitude to medication • Parental separation	• Therapy offered in groups to contain costs • Therapist urges further evidence-based treatment (p)
Current	• ADHD • Anxiety disorder	• Ongoing family turmoil heightens anxiety/inattention • Declining self-esteem	• School performance deteriorates • Custody battle • Lost to follow-up mental health care	

FIGURE 8.1. Formulation grid for Malcolm.

for attentional difficulties, but one often criticized by the North American media), Malcolm's mother insisted on an anxiety-focused assessment. She also blamed the teacher for her son's academic difficulties and disagreed with her husband's view that Malcolm had no problems, resulting in Malcolm receiving very mixed messages from the adults in his life. Such mixed messages would probably have reduced his motivation to improve his schoolwork. Inconsistency among parents with respect to behavior management (given their disagreement as to the nature of his difficulties) may also have exacerbated Malcolm's inattentive symptoms.

Malcolm's psychiatric assessment concluded that he suffered from both ADHD and an anxiety disorder, and the evidence-based treatment for both disorders was recommended. However, given the societal need to contain health care costs, the anxiety-focused therapy was offered in a group format. Given Malcolm's high distractibility and learning difficulties, the expectation that he learn coping strategies for managing his anxiety in a group was unrealistic, especially given the lack of medication to ameliorate his inattention. The evidence-based treatment for ADHD was refused by Malcolm's mother, probably due to cultural bias against using psychotropic medication in children, thus perpetuating Malcolm's distractibility and related school problems. Meanwhile, Malcolm's ongoing learning difficulties and school failure were likely having adverse effects on his self-esteem and his optimism regarding future school success, reducing motivation to learn. Failure to benefit from therapy reinforced this lack of optimism and motivation. The therapist, appropriately, recommended additional treatment but did not have the opportunity to ensure it was implemented.

The separation of Malcolm's parents almost certainly heightened his anxiety, as is common in children of his age. Family turmoil around the separation would have exacerbated both inattention and anxiety. Thus, his school performance would now be affected by a combination of inattention, anxiety, family disorganization, and motivational factors, resulting in further deterioration. The custody battle between Malcolm's parents subsequently reduced the chances of further educational remediation or further mental health follow-up. Malcolm's prognosis for academic success and a return to healthy emotional development is therefore bleak.

IMPORTANT CONSIDERATIONS IN SCHOOL-AGE CHILDREN

The following is a list of key points from previous chapters that highlight important considerations when constructing formulations for school-age children.

- Constitutional abilities and vulnerabilities (e.g,. difficult temperament, medical illnesses and their treatments) become more noticeable as children face the challenges associated with school entry.
- Children with emotional problems may present with somatic symptoms (e.g., stomachaches or headaches) at this age.
- Comparisons with peers in school settings are inevitable and sometimes result in stigmatization of children with physical or developmental disabilities.
- Children's interpretations of illness may focus on its effects on competence/school performance and on fear of mutilation/loss of bodily integrity.
- Chronic illness may affect children's level of independence from family.
- Realistic view of death as permanent (starting at about age 8) can produce anxiety.
- School-age children have a greater vocabulary for feelings than preschoolers.
- School-age children can take others' points of view, attend to more than one dimension at a time, and find solutions to realistic problems (sometimes with assistance).
- School-age children have an emerging ability to separate thoughts, feelings, and behaviors and see connections among them (mental phenomena are still seen in concrete ways, though).
- Parents still need to support/scaffold regulation of feelings in children at this age.
- Accomplishment (e.g., academic, athletic, life skills) is a psychological focus at this age, as is following the rules at home and at school.
- Inattention and other neuropsychological problems interfere with these foci.
- Adjusting to various aspects of school can become a source of stress/difficulty.
- Family–school relationships can be challenging.
- Family expectations regarding school accomplishment and/or various ethnic/cultural/religious activities can sometimes be stressful for children.
- Friendships and peer acceptance become increasingly important to the child.
- Bullying can have significant adverse effects on mental health.
- Family attitudes toward peers and the larger community can

limit or enhance children's opportunities for social experiences.

- Many children at this age have had prior mental health contacts, which may affect the child's and family's expectations of the clinician.
- Familial and cultural attitudes toward mental health intervention may delay or prevent treatment in some cases.
- Media and other cultural influences may affect children's emerging self-concept and values
- Community supports are important to mitigate the stresses faced by many young families.
- Cultural expectations regarding the child's behavior, childrearing practices, and mental illness and its treatment are important to explore with families regardless of child age.
- To engage in treatment, children of this age are still dependent on their families' acceptance of North American ideas about mental health care (see example of Jorge in Chapter 6).
- Children's spiritual concepts are still fairly concrete at this age, often focused on stories and rules, and usually consistent with those of their families.
- Spiritually based coping and support from communities of faith are potential protective factors in children of all ages.

FURTHER EXAMPLES OF CASE FORMULATION

To gain experience doing case formulation in this age group, let's revisit the examples of Abby, a 10-year-old girl with a seizure disorder described in Chapter 3, and Serena, an 11-year-old girl with severe oppositionality described in Chapter 4. Use the steps listed in Chapter 7. That is, for each case try to create a formulation grid with arrows to indicate related factors. Then, write the case formulation as a story. Figures 8.2 and 8.3 show sample formulation grids for Abby and Serena (respectively), and one possible case formulation for each is written below.

Interestingly, Abby's case illustrates that the interaction of various factors does not always result in the child "going from bad to worse" as occurred with Malcolm. In the second half of Abby's case, the interaction of several protective factors serves to ameliorate previous problems. As a result, Abby's relationship with her mother improves, her anxiety decreases, and she returns to a mentally healthy developmental trajectory with good seizure control. This case provides an important example of how building upon protective factors can form the basis of very successful interventions.

Serena's case, on the other hand, shows a different pattern. In this case, many risk factors converge on a single outcome: poor regulation of emotions and mistrust of others. As described in Chapter 1, developmental psychologists refer to this phenomenon as "equifinality." Any one of Serena's risk factors could contribute to poor emotional control, but the cumulative effect of all of them over the course of development leaves Serena in a very emotionally unstable state. There are some protective factors, which could be built upon in treatment, but they have not yet had a significant impact on Serena's development. The opposite pattern, "multifinality," can also be seen sometimes. In this case, a single risk or protective factor can lead to many different outcomes. For example, intelligence can result in school success and therefore heightened self-esteem and emotional health. However, in a culture in which "book-learning" is not valued, intelligence can result in a child becoming unpopular and ostracized among peers, which can be damaging to emotional health. In summary, each risk or protective factor contributes little to predicting a child's ultimate developmental outcome, but by understanding the interactions among factors over time we can see more clearly how various outcomes emerge.

Case Example: Abby (see Figure 8.2)

Until age 10, Abby was the physically and mentally healthy daughter of a single mother who had a history of anxiety. At that age, Abby suddenly developed seizures. The fact that the initial treating physician minimized the concerns of Abby's mother heightened her anxiety, as did the struggle to find effective anti-seizure medication for Abby. This anxiety about her child likely resulted in a somewhat overprotective parenting style in Abby's mother.

Once effective anti-seizure medication was found, it caused mild cognitive impairment in Abby. The seizures, the adverse effect of the cognitive impairment on her school performance, and her mother's anxiety and overprotection all likely increased Abby's anxiety. Maternal anxiety would likely be transmitted via both genetic factors and the mother's modeling of anxious coping. The anxiety in both mother and child, ongoing school struggles, and the ongoing need to manage Abby's seizures (with both medication and adequate sleep) all

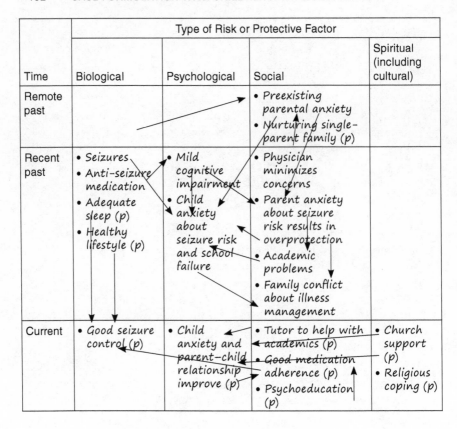

Time	Type of Risk or Protective Factor			
	Biological	Psychological	Social	Spiritual (including cultural)
Remote past			• Preexisting parental anxiety • Nurturing single-parent family (p)	
Recent past	• Seizures • Anti-seizure medication • Adequate sleep (p) • Healthy lifestyle (p)	• Mild cognitive impairment • Child anxiety about seizure risk and school failure	• Physician minimizes concerns • Parent anxiety about seizure risk results in overprotection • Academic problems • Family conflict about illness management	
Current	• Good seizure control (p)	• Child anxiety and parent–child relationship improve (p)	• Tutor to help with academics (p) • Good medication adherence (p) • Psychoeducation (p)	• Church support (p) • Religious coping (p)

FIGURE 8.2. Formulation grid for Abby.

contributed to family conflict. Such conflict would be detrimental to both school success and seizure control.

Fortunately, Abby and her mother responded well to mental health intervention and spiritual support. They were able to benefit from psychoeducation about the nature of Abby's illness and its management, were able to engage a tutor to reduce academic stress, and were open to assistance from their church, which provided both community support and religious coping. All of these protective factors reduced tension in the parent–child relationship, which resulted in better medication adherence, reduced anxiety in Abby and her mother, better school performance, and Abby's return to a mentally healthy course of development. Abby's healthy lifestyle, good sleep routines, and good medication adherence in turn improved seizure control, improving her physical health as well.

Case Example: Serena (see Figure 8.3)

Serena's early difficult temperament, language-based learning disability, possible ADHD, and her mother's depression may represent biologically based, constitutional vulnerabilities to poor emotion regulation and mental health difficulties. Both language and the ability to focus are important to the development of higher-level cognitive abilities, which are needed to regulate feelings. Maternal depression represents both a genetic vulnerability factor and an environmental one in this case, as it is frequently associated with insecure attachment when it

Time	Type of Risk or Protective Factor			
	Biological	Psychological	Social	Spiritual (including cultural)
Remote past	• Difficult temperament • Language-based learning disability • Possible ADHD	• Maternal postpartum depression • Probable attachment insecurity • Possibly witnessed domestic violence	• High-conflict family • Inconsistent behavior management	
Recent past	"	• Failure to keep up at school lowers self-esteem • Development of self-control and trust lagging • Anxiety limits oppositional behavior at school but not home	• School and parents expect her to demonstrate conceptual reasoning	• Limited access to community activities and treatments (family suspicion)
Current	"	• Mistrust of authority • Low motivation to succeed • Engages with therapist, but superficially • Seeks attention by acting out	• Socially adept with peers (p) • School community is helpful (not punitive) (p)	• Allowed to access treatment (p)

FIGURE 8.3. Formulation grid for Serena.

occurs in the postpartum period. Insecure attachment, in turn, impairs the development of higher-level cognitive abilities (see Chapter 7). Family conflict and especially witnessing domestic violence would be emotionally disturbing to Serena, further impairing her self-regulation ability. Many parents of children who misbehave learn to calmly and consistently manage the behavior, resulting in improvement. The inconsistency between Serena's parents and their continued conflict impeded this process, resulting in worsening behavior over time.

Starting school highlighted Serena's learning and attention deficits when compared to other children. Her inability to trust authority figures, such as teachers (likely related to insecure attachment to parents), prevented Serena from accessing academic help. Lack of success at school was stressful; it resulted in increased behavioral problems at home, and it began to adversely affect her self-esteem as she repeatedly failed to meet adult expectations regarding her learning and behavior. School behavior was relatively contained by Serena's anxiety about getting into trouble, representing a protective factor in this case. The inability of Serena's parents to trust each other, or therapists, or other community members reduced Serena's access to helpful activities or treatments that might have otherwise improved her self-esteem, level of trust, and ability to regulate feelings.

By the time she presented at the consultation, Serena's lack of school success and low self-esteem had resulted in learned helplessness (i.e., giving up before starting academic work), undermining her motivation. Furthermore, her chronic inability to regulate her feelings had caused habitual attention-seeking behavior. For Serena, acting out had become a way of engaging adults in her emotional turmoil and was becoming a way of life. Moreover, Serena's attachment-related mistrust of authority figures had led to unsuccessful, superficial therapeutic relationships with mental health professionals, even when her parents were willing to allow these to be involved. Nevertheless, Serena's ability to relate to her peers with humor, her sympathetic school environment, and her parents' recent attempts to cooperate for her benefit represent potential protective factors that merit further attention and development.

The examples in this chapter have highlighted a few of the struggles of the school-age child and provided a chance to practice the process of case formulation as outlined in Chapter 7. This process will become more challenging, but hopefully also more interesting, as we consider the complexities of adolescence in Chapter 9.

Case Formulation for Adolescents

The psychology of adolescence builds upon all previous developmental tasks, often resulting in rich and complex case formulations in this age group. Identity formation, however, is a central theme and so receives additional attention in this chapter. Key developmental considerations from previous chapters are also reviewed, and three case examples are provided to illustrate different adolescent mental health challenges. To start, however, it is important to acknowledge that eliciting accurate and complete information from adolescents is not always easy. Therefore, key aspects of communication with adolescents are highlighted below.

COMMUNICATING WITH ADOLESCENTS

Like a parent, a clinician assessing an adolescent is often regarded with suspicion. Failure to respect the adolescent's emerging need for autonomy is particularly likely to result in a breakdown of communication. For example, telling an adolescent "I suggest you do this" may elicit skepticism ("Why should I do it?") or even hostility ("You can't make me do it!") By contrast, an indirect comment such as "I wonder if this is a possibility" may be received more favorably, resulting in the adolescent considering the suggestion. Similarly, trying to express empathy for a teen by saying, "That must be hard" may be misinterpreted as telling him or her what to think or feel and therefore result in rejection. Asking the question "How is that for you?," although the answer may be obvious, often seems more respectful and empathic to the teen. Asking for adolescents' agreement or participation may also alienate them. For example, "Let's look this up online, OK?" may elicit a yawn. However, if the clinician says, "I think I'll look that up online" and pulls up an extra chair, the adolescent may eventually join in.

Other ideas to keep in mind when talking with adolescents or their parents include:

- Adolescents sometimes need to feign invincibility in order to feel autonomous. Challenging their bravado is rarely helpful, unless they are planning something dangerous.
- Adolescents are typically very self-conscious and reluctant to talk about feeling embarrassed. Talking about what others said or did in relation to the teen is often more effective than commenting on the embarrassment.
- Adolescents often need more parental help than they are willing to acknowledge, but it is often wise to introduce this topic with "What do you want your parents to do?" rather than "What do you need your parents to do?"
- Adolescents often minimize the importance of family versus peers, so talking about peers first and family later can be helpful.
- Adolescents are often more comfortable talking about facts or experiences than feelings (as talking about feelings makes most people feel vulnerable).
- Talking about peers as "people in your class" or "your friends" is usually preferable to talking about "other kids" or "other teens," as the latter may seem disrespectful of peers.
- When in doubt, listen to the adolescent rather than give advice.
- It is important to be clear about the limits of confidentiality with teens (i.e., dangerous situations will always be reported), but in the absence of danger, teens should be able to tell clinicians what they do or do not want their parents to know, and their wishes should generally be respected.
- Clinicians should try *not* to take sides when teens and parents disagree, as siding with the teen can create the false expectation that the clinician will convince the parents to change and siding with the parents can alienate the teen. Problem solving with teens about how to cope with their parents' demands (and

assuming these are not going to change) is usually more productive.

- Parents of teens often feel helpless, as they cannot control their adolescents' behavior. Talking to parents about their importance as role models and their ability to *influence* (rather than control) behavior is often helpful. Books such as *How to Talk So Teens Will Listen and Listen So Teens Will Talk* (Faber & Mazlish, 2005) can also be recommended.

ADOLESCENT IDENTITY FORMATION

Development of one's individual identity is a key developmental task of adolescence. Some authors consider this task as a two-step process: (1) psychological separation from one's family of origin (i.e., adolescence as "the second separation–individuation"; Blos, 1979) and (2) developing a stable, cohesive sense of one's self. In most cases, however, the two steps occur concurrently, and the progression between the two steps is not necessarily smooth. More often, both autonomy and a sense of one's self go "two steps forward, one step back." For example, it is not unusual for young teens to appear very autonomous from their families of origin for a time and then regress to a more dependent state when faced with a stressful event such as starting high school.

When doing case formulation, however, it is often helpful to think of the two steps separately, as autonomy relates more to family interactions (i.e., a social aspect of the case formulation) and a sense of self relates more to psychological aspects of the case formulation. Within the family, problematic cycles of interaction can develop around an adolescent's struggle for autonomy. Some examples include the following:

1. A parent worries about an adolescent who appears secretive, but the adolescent may become annoyed with his intrusive parent and withdraw, prompting further parental concern.
2. A parent gets frustrated about an adolescent's lack of participation in family activities and therefore criticizes the teen, but the teen then withdraws in order to avoid the criticism, causing more parental frustration.
3. A worried parent may provide excessive reassurance to an adolescent who appears anxious about independence, undermining

his or her confidence and thus further reducing attempts at independent behavior.

4. An overburdened parent may withdraw from an anxious adolescent's requests for support, leaving the adolescent feeling more anxious and resulting in more requests for support.

Even though these examples of interaction cycles appear to begin with the parent, each can also begin with the adolescent, and by the time the clinician observes them it is usually not possible to determine with whom they started. Moreover, the patterns may differ between the adolescent and each parent or even alternate within the same relationship over time. They occur in most parent–adolescent relationships to some degree, and it is the extent of their interference with adolescent development that determines how healthy or unhealthy they are considered to be.

Parents of adolescents often express particular concerns about their children's identification with peers. One fear they commonly describe is that their teen will succumb to peer pressure and become involved with illicit drugs or other unsavory activities. Parents may be tempted to intrude upon their teen's privacy (e.g., searching his or her room) in order to reassure themselves. Unfortunately, this attitude usually results in family interaction pattern 1 just described, with the teen disclosing progressively less information to parents about his or her peer activities. It is sometimes helpful to understand (and help parents understand) that, developmentally, identifying with one's peer group often serves as a stepping-stone toward true autonomy from one's family of origin. Moreover, identification with peers can have positive as well as negative consequences. For example, therapeutic groups with adolescents often rely on positive peer influences to encourage courageous behavior (in the case of anxious teens) or promote increased levels of activity (in the case of depressed teens). Peers in school clubs that focus on environmental issues or other social causes can similarly exert a positive influence on teens. Therefore, rather than asking parents "Are you concerned that your teen may be influenced by peers?" it is often more fruitful to ask "Do you know who your teen's friends are and what they like to do as a group?" Teens who trust their parents enough to tell them about peer activities usually feel supported at home, reducing the chances that they will compromise their values to please their peer group.

As reviewed in Chapter 4, developing a cohesive sense of self can represent either a culmination of previous developmental tasks or an opportunity for developmental reorganization. In the first case, the child arrives at adolescence able to explore new challenges from the "secure base" of attachment to one or more dependable adults, clear psychological boundaries between himself and others, enough self-worth to express herself without fearing shame or humiliation, a healthy self-discipline, and the ability to pursue his or her interests diligently without excessive fear of failure. Building upon these personal and interpersonal strengths, the adolescent is in a very good position to negotiate the challenges of individuation and identity formation. On the other hand, Perdita (described in Chapter 6) provides a glimpse of identity formation as an opportunity for developmental reorganization. In this case, a young woman with poor psychological boundaries in relation to her critical, demanding mother becomes quite self-critical, resulting in a number of psychiatric symptoms. In adolescence, she overcomes this unhealthy interpersonal pattern through belief in a comforting God who does not expect the complete acquiescence her mother demands. As she becomes more accepting of herself and her own imperfections, her symptoms decline. One would predict that over time Perdita's more self-accepting attitude would also allow for more authentic relationships with others and clearer interpersonal boundaries.

The results of adolescent struggles have been categorized by identity theorist James Marcia (1966). Marcia identified four possible states of identity development in adolescents with respect to values and ideals, sexual orientation, and vocational goals. They are not intended to be stages that involve progression from one state to the next, but rather four possible ways that an adolescent may be dealing with the challenge of identity formation. These states are sometimes useful when formulating adolescent responses to this challenge. They include the following: identity achievement, in which an individual has made the commitments needed to build a sense of identity after coming through a period of exploration and uncertainty; foreclosure, in which a commitment to a particular occupation or life path has been made without exploring a range of options; identity diffusion, in which the youth has not made a commitment to any particular long-term goal or identity and is not currently trying to do so; and moratorium, in which the adolescent is actively exploring a range of options, but has not made a decision yet.

Marcia's four states imply that identity formation ought to include a period of exploration and uncertainty, rather than prematurely accepting a life path that has not been well considered or has been chosen by others for the youth. For example, Fatima in Chapter 6 was a young

Muslim woman who went through considerable soul searching as she tried to balance her parents' wish to have her blend in with the local population and her own desire to stand out from the crowd in a positive way. Eventually, she decided to wear traditional Muslim attire even though her parents initially disapproved and she was uncertain how her peers would react. Asserting her autonomy in this way was a risk, but one that ultimately had very positive results for Fatima. By contrast, Robert (also from Chapter 6) was an intelligent but aimless young man from an impoverished and emotionally rejecting background. When a charismatic gang leader paid attention to him, Robert readily adopted an identity as a gang member without much consideration of the consequences. This choice would be considered a "foreclosure" solution, with very unfortunate results. The state of foreclosure can also occur with respect to identity options that are considered socially acceptable or even laudable. For example, in my own peer group of adolescents whose parents were first-generation immigrants, many chose career options their families expected (e.g., physicians, dentists, lawyers) with little exploration of alternatives. Several later changed careers or expressed disappointment with their choices.

Marcia's theory emphasizes values and ideals, sexual orientation, and vocational goals as important aspects of identity. However, many other aspects have been cited as important in adolescent development by other authors. In fact, there are several aspects of identity one could consider with respect to each of the main aspects of case formulation (biological, psychological, social, and spiritual/cultural). These aspects are shown in Table 9.1. It is worth reviewing this table when formulating adolescent cases, as uncertainty or discomfort in any of these areas can cause adolescents distress and therefore result in psychological symptoms.

Rather than merely labeling the teen's difficulty, however, it is important to examine potential developmental antecedents that may be contributing to the problem. By revisiting the example of Paul (from Chapter 2), a young teen with depression and cannabis abuse, we can see how a number of developmental influences were at play in forming his self-described interpersonal identity of "I am trouble." Paul's formulation grid is presented in Figure 9.1 with arrows indicating connections among different factors. As shown, the factors contributing to his "troubled" identity included lack of achievement at school, likely related to his ADHD traits; association with antisocial peers, likely related to his mistrust of authority figures (stemming from insecure attachment) and lack of reliable parental support (stemming from

TABLE 9.1. Biological, Psychological, Social, and Spiritual/Cultural Aspects of Identity

Biological domain

- Body image
- Gender identity
- Athletic ability
- Attractiveness

Psychological domain

- Occupation
- Cognitive ability
- Interests
- Self-esteem ("How worthy am I?")
- Self-concept ("What are my strengths and weaknesses?")
- Psychological boundaries
- Interpersonal expectations of self and others

Social domain

- Sexual orientation
- Collective/group identity
- Interpersonal identity (e.g., "What sort of friend, student, daughter/son, sister/brother, leader am I?")

Spiritual/cultural domain

- Values
- Religious/spiritual beliefs
- Ethnic/cultural identity

marital conflict and different parenting styles); being disliked by teachers, likely related to his mistrust of authority figures, antisocial peer associations, and lack of achievement at school; and finally the lack of reliable parental support itself, which prevented either parent from effectively encouraging a more positive interpersonal identity.

The following account is one possible formulation of Paul's case that highlights the central role of this identity:

Paul was a temperamentally active, possibly hyperactive youngster who was born into a highly conflicted marriage characterized by cultural and personality contrasts. His father's unavailability and his mother's resentment of him (due to the similarity between Paul and his father) prevented either parent from providing Paul with reliable support and encouragement, resulting in Paul developing an insecure attachment style and mistrust of authority figures. His parents' opposing, inconsistent behavior management styles further exacerbated

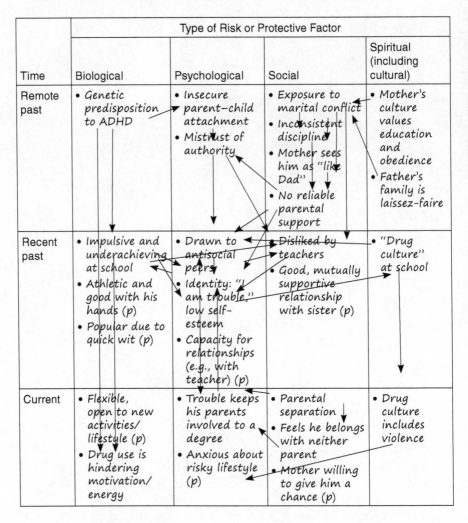

FIGURE 9.1. Revisiting the formulation grid for Paul.

Paul's disruptive behavior. Given his insecurity and ongoing behavior problems, Paul began considering himself a troublemaker within his family.

Upon starting school, Paul's mistrust of authority, disruptive behavior, and association with antisocial peers (whom he trusted more than adults, given his home life) made him a troublemaker in the eyes of his teachers as well. As he delved more deeply into the anti-social, drug-using lifestyle, Paul increasingly came to see himself as his teachers did, and his self-esteem declined. Whether he was aware of it or not, Paul's ongoing behavior problems and "trouble" identity also kept his parents involved in his life, eliciting a small amount of support from them and perhaps preventing their eventual separation for a time.

As his family broke up and ongoing drug use exacerbated his school difficulties, Paul's view of himself as an unlikable troublemaker intensified, and he became increasingly depressed. Despite his athleticism, dexterity, humor, and capacity for relationships (demonstrated in those with his sister and his shop teacher), Paul's view of himself persisted. It did not change significantly until drug-related violence made both Paul and his mother anxious enough about his lifestyle to seek and participate in treatment.

IMPORTANT DEVELOPMENTAL CONSIDERATIONS IN ADOLESCENCE

The following list highlights key points from Chapters 3–6 pertaining to adolescent development:

- Adolescents' ability to "think about thinking" (called formal operations) is conducive to psychotherapy, but engagement in therapy may be challenging owing to adolescent autonomy needs.
- Abstract, hypothetical reasoning develops in most adolescents, but their social judgment often lags behind.
- Heightened self-consciousness is common in this age group (e.g., the "imaginary audience").
- Adolescents become increasingly self-reliant in regulating their feelings but still need parental guidance and support.
- Responses to illness in this age group may focus on the condition's effects on body image, effects on peer relationships, effects on autonomy (including rebelling against treatment), concerns about effects on intimate relationships, and concerns about implications for long-term goals.
- Engagement in and adherence to treatment is increasingly within the adolescent's control, rather than being dictated by the family.
- Pubertal hormonal changes can exacerbate some conditions

differentially by gender (e.g., heightened anxiety and depression in postpubertal girls).

- Substance abuse should be suspected if there is a new onset of cognitive impairment or psychiatric symptoms.
- Interpersonal patterns emerge in adolescence and can be examined with the young person; sometimes these are due to adolescents' expectations of themselves or others that relate to old attachment patterns.
- Developing one's identity and independence from one's family of origin is a major psychological focus of adolescence.
- Intimate relationships and sexuality start to become a focus in adolescence but continue into adulthood.
- Adolescents are often appearance conscious, so physical differences become more concerning at this age.
- Adolescents oscillate between dependence and independence from family, and some families cope better with this behavior than others.
- Adolescents can experience tension between emerging personal values and family values.
- Peer, media, and web influences become more salient in adolescence and may conflict with family values but may also be a source of meaning (adolescent activism regarding the environment, child labor, etc.).
- Family attitudes toward peers and the larger community can limit or enhance adolescents' opportunities for social experiences.
- Many teens have had prior mental health contacts, which may affect the adolescent and family's expectations of the clinician.
- Community supports are important to mitigate the stresses faced by many families regardless of child age.
- Pressure to succeed academically can increase as teens prepare for postsecondary education.
- Cultural expectations regarding the child's behavior, childrearing practices, and mental illness and its treatment are important to explore with families regardless of child age.
- Adolescents' spiritual concepts are increasingly abstract and not always consistent with those of their families.
- Values and beliefs are an important aspect of adolescent identity, as is cultural or ethnic identity.
- Spiritually based coping and support from communities of faith are potential protective factors in children of all ages.

FURTHER EXAMPLES OF CASE FORMULATION FOR ADOLESCENTS

The case formulation for Paul earlier in this chapter emphasized the role of adolescent identity. In some cases, however, identity is still in flux, but certain patterns of coping are becoming increasingly habitual and entrenched. Biologically, this makes sense as brain circuits are modified throughout development according to the "use it or lose it" principle. In other words, connections among brain cells that are used repeatedly become more efficient, and those that are neglected are eventually lost. Thus, by adolescence, the range of thinking and coping patterns used is gradually decreasing relative to the range of patterns used by a younger child. Interactions between nature and nurture, between the child's temperament and environmental influences, are slowly becoming less malleable and, by age 18, are considered personality traits. The remaining two examples illustrate maladaptive coping styles in adolescents that will require substantial intervention to change.

Case Example: Raj (see Figure 9.2)

Coping with stressful situations by avoiding them is a common pattern in anxious youth. These teens have developed a sense of personal helplessness, often over years, and are therefore ill equipped to face the challenges of adolescence. Raj, a 15-year-old boy with long-standing school avoidance, illustrates this coping pattern.

Raj was born at 7 months' gestation, the youngest of three children in an intact family. Raj required life support initially because of his prematurity. Fortunately, he made progress rapidly and was soon meeting his developmental milestones. However, he often had bouts of asthma requiring emergency visits in the toddler and preschool years, resulting in his parents always considering him a "sickly" child. He was also noted to have a somewhat rigid temperament, becoming easily upset when daily routines were changed even slightly. He was also sensitive to certain fabrics and certain food textures. He tended to be perfectionistic and criticized peers who did not follow the rules but was able to make friends and was otherwise socially appropriate.

Raj's father was a successful businessman who engaged in frequent work-related travel. He had dropped out of high school owing to symptoms of ADHD and believed that "book smarts" were not nearly as valuable as the ability to work hard and "make connections" with others. Raj's mother worked at home to raise her children. She had

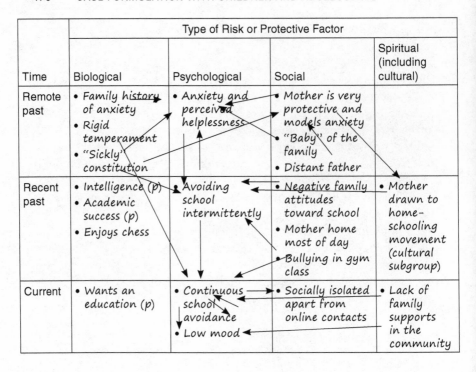

FIGURE 9.2. Formulation grid for Raj.

a history of panic disorder and, although able to leave the house for errands, she did not drive.

Raj began missing school intermittently in the elementary years, often following a cold or "flu," when he tended to be absent for several weeks. His mother would look after Raj at home, read him stories, and not insist he return to school as long as he reported stomachaches or other discomfort. When challenged about this practice by a teacher, she reported that her "baby" was not ready to return to the "rough" peer group at his school and needed time to heal. She began associating with a group of women who were homeschooling their children or advocating this practice. The family had no connections to other families or other community organizations. Nevertheless, Raj showed obvious intelligence and seemed to enjoy school. He did well academically, sometimes winning academic awards, and excelled in the chess club.

Soon after starting high school at age 14, Raj experienced a distressing incident in gym class. He had difficulty lifting a weight that his peers were hoisting easily and was embarrassed. After class, one of his peers called him a name implying that he was homosexual, and the other boys joined in the name-calling. Raj was not yet dating but self-identified as heterosexual. He was deeply humiliated by the incident and did not return to school after that day.

Raj's mother felt it was the school's responsibility to ensure an environment where her son would feel safe, but the school's efforts to address the peer problems over the course of the following year were never sufficient in her eyes. She indicated a preference for homeschooling her son. Raj's father had a distant relationship with his son and stated that in his experience school was "useless" and the boy should get a job. Raj was hoping to return to school, stating that he wanted an education, "unlike my ignorant Dad." However, he reported feeling anxious about going back and did not think this was possible until he felt better. Medical and psychological treatment for anxiety was initiated, but several months later Raj still did not feel ready to return "until I am 100%." He spent his days playing video games on his computer and communicating with friends via the Internet. His communications took on an increasingly negative tone. Whenever he was urged to return to school, Raj began hyperventilating with anxiety and sometimes threatened to harm himself.

In Figure 9.2, some of the connections among Raj's risk factors for chronic school avoidance are shown, and will now be formulated. There are some biological protective factors as well (intelligence, academic success, enjoys chess, wants an education), but Raj has not been able to use these protective measures to overcome his difficulty. Nevertheless, they are worth keeping in mind when planning treatment (see Chapter 11, pp. 209–210).

Raj's development of an avoidant coping style that interferes with school attendance derives from multiple factors. His family history of anxiety, "sickly" constitution (whether actually present or merely perceived by his family), maternal protectiveness and modeling of anxiety (intensified by his father's frequent absences), and ordinal position as the youngest ("baby") in the family all predispose to anxiety and the perception of himself as a relatively helpless, dependent individual. His intermittent school avoidance following minor illnesses would reinforce this perception of himself. Illness in Raj would also heighten his mother's anxiety, causing her to focus on his vulnerability, his "rough" peers, and the option of homeschooling. The latter philosophy also provided the family's only connection to the larger community, increasing its impact. Both parents' negative attitudes toward school and the fact that Raj's mother did not work outside the home also facilitated intermittent absenteeism.

The taunting by Raj's peers in gym class was cruel and clearly triggered his continuous absenteeism. Humiliating incidents are particularly difficult to overcome for youth with perfectionistic tendencies like Raj. His rigid, perfectionistic temperament also prevented Raj from attempting a return to school until he felt "100%." However, all of the factors that contributed to Raj's intermittent absenteeism also perpetuated his ongoing school avoidance. With prolonged school avoidance, decreased social contact, and decreased opportunities for accomplishment, Raj's self-esteem declined and his mood plummeted. His depressed mood further reduced his motivation to return to school. In the face of Raj's suicidal threats, his parents' ambivalence about school, and their lack of supports outside the family, the chances of Raj's parents successfully facilitating school return were very slim.

Practitioners might wonder what will happen to Raj. One possibility is that his depression will become more severe, eventually warranting more intensive treatment and alerting his parents to the need to change their attitudes. However, this sort of crisis does not always occur in cases of chronic school avoidance. In the absence of a crisis, family interactions that have been present for years are often self-perpetuating and difficult to change, particularly as teens reach an age at which school attendance is no longer compulsory. Perhaps Raj's own statement regarding his "ignorant Dad" offers a glimmer of hope. It shows an emerging desire for autonomy from parents and a young man who values getting an education. These developmentally appropriate goals may eventually increase Raj's own motivation sufficiently to prompt a return to school or to another educational path (e.g., correspondence courses). However, he will likely need additional mental health interventions to overcome his unhealthy, avoidant coping style and reach his full potential.

Case Example: Dawn (see Figure 9.3)

Unlike Raj, some adolescents do not appear to have a consistent preferred coping style. Rather, they seem to be "grasping at straws" whenever they encounter stressful situations and use multiple unhealthy means of trying to regulate negative emotions. Over time, however, this chronic emotional instability can become a pattern too and predispose the teen to personality disorders in adulthood, particularly borderline personality disorder. Dawn is a young woman who illustrates

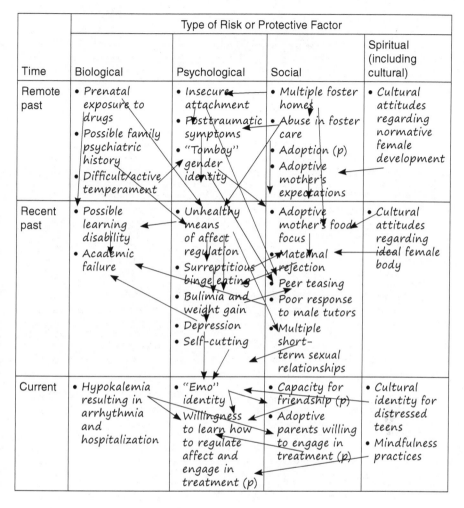

FIGURE 9.3. Formulation grid for Dawn.

this pattern. Her rather complicated case formulation is illustrated in Figure 9.3.

Dawn was a heavyset girl of 17 with a short, boyish haircut who presented to the emergency room after losing consciousness briefly. She was found to have an arrhythmia (irregular heartbeat) due to a very low level of potassium in her bloodstream. When questioned, she admitted to frequent self-induced vomiting in order to control her weight. Her low potassium and resulting irregular heartbeat were consequences of this behavior. Dawn had presented to the emergency room several times before with nonlethal self-injurious behavior. Her forearms were covered in scars from superficial self-inflicted cuts. She often begged to be admitted to the hospital but then left against medical advice within a day or two, so she was now routinely discharged from the emergency room once her medical condition was stable. Dawn was sometimes accompanied by a boy or a girl whom she identified as her partner. She had engaged in numerous short-term sexual relationships and self-identified as bisexual, but her longest relationship had lasted 4 months.

Dawn's early history was difficult and traumatic. Dawn's mother had used several illicit drugs during her pregnancy, and Dawn suffered withdrawal symptoms at birth. Her father had spent time in a psychiatric facility, but his exact diagnosis was not known. He had never been involved in Dawn's life. Given the unfortunate circumstances of her birth, Dawn was removed from her mother's care and placed in foster care. She lived in eight different foster homes before the age of 7, when she was adopted by an older, childless couple. Unfortunately, she was sexually abused at age 3 in one of her foster placements, but these traumatic experiences had never been addressed therapeutically. Although Dawn suffered from bedwetting and recurrent nightmares, her adoptive mother indicated that she did not believe in "dredging up the past."

Dawn's adoptive mother had always wanted a daughter and dressed her "like a princess." Dawn was an active youngster, however, and disliked her frilly clothes and carefully coiffed hairstyles. She preferred T-shirts and jeans. In grade 5, much to her mother's chagrin, Dawn cut her hair in the school bathroom with scissors she was using for an art project. Trying to channel Dawn's need for activity in a positive way, her adoptive mother decided to enroll her in ballet. Dawn hated ballet, but she cooperated as she craved parental attention and approval.

Academically, Dawn was struggling to keep up. She could read but often reversed her letters when she was writing and misunderstood instructions in math and other subjects. Dawn's parents enrolled her in a private elementary school, where children with learning difficulties were supported with extra help and academic expectations were modest. There was no private high school near Dawn's home, however, so she switched to the public system in grade 9.

When Dawn reached puberty, her adoptive mother began monitoring her food intake closely, as Dawn could not be fat if she was going to succeed in ballet. Dawn responded by secretly consuming junk food. When Dawn's adoptive mother found her "sneaking" food or otherwise behaving in ways considered unladylike, she deliberately ignored her daughter. Dawn would apologize profusely but be met with silence. Feeling rejected, she ate more food to comfort herself. Occasionally, she also took a razor blade to her arm in an attempt to punish herself.

Moreover, Dawn's academic problems became more severe as expectations at her high school were far greater than those at her sheltered private school had been. Dawn's parents arranged for tutoring, but unfortunately with a series of male tutors. Dawn responded negatively to each of them. As she became more discouraged with school and more alienated from her adoptive mother, Dawn's mood also became worse. Peer teasing about her ballooning weight exacerbated her mood further and left her fatigued and unmotivated at school.

Self-induced vomiting seemed to be one means of controlling her weight and maintaining her mother's approval. Without that approval, Dawn described herself as "empty." She had also discovered that cutting her arms seemed to temporarily relieve some emotional distress and so began engaging in this behavior regularly. Sexual relationships also made her feel less "empty," and she found herself drawn toward partners of either gender. Dawn's adoptive parents were embarrassed by her behavior and responded by distancing themselves from her.

Dawn's repeated emergency visits and academic failure alienated her from many peers, until she met a group of misfits at school who self-identified as "Emo" (emotionally disturbed). They wore dark clothing, did not participate in school activities, and sometimes got into trouble for spraying negative graffiti messages on the school walls. Dawn felt a kinship with them and began associating with this group. One girl in the group was diagnosed with depression and started to learn some mindfulness practices from her therapist. Dawn had joined her a few times and found this helpful.

After the incident in which she lost consciousness, Dawn was admitted to a medical floor of the hospital. She was told she was lucky to be alive and had to remain in the hospital for a week to have her heart monitored. Frightened, she agreed to psychiatric treatment, which involved both individual therapy and family therapy with her adoptive parents. Recognizing the gravity of the situation, her adoptive parents agreed too.

When reading Dawn's story, some of the reasons for her problems may be obvious to most mental health practitioners. However, given the number of risk factors in this case and the complexity of their interrelationships, formulating Dawn's case is daunting. If such complexity is daunting for the practitioner, though, how much more daunting must it be for a teen like Dawn who is living with this emotional chaos! Dawn's story serves as a sobering reminder that shunning or ridiculing emotionally disturbed youth is never appropriate. When someone encounters as many developmental challenges as Dawn has, expecting a normative outcome may not be realistic.

Rather than attempting to connect all of the ways in which Dawn's development went awry, let's summarize some key links among factors. These include the following:

- Prenatal drug exposure can predispose children to both learning disabilities and impaired emotion regulation, both of which can contribute to academic failure.
- Insecure attachment is a very common result of placement in multiple foster homes.
- Insecure attachment and traumatic experiences can both interfere with the development of emotion regulation.
- Sexual abuse likely contributed to ongoing posttraumatic symptoms, mistrust of males, and poor emotion regulation in this case, and may have affected gender identity and sexual orientation (note: constitutional factors often play a role in the latter two outcomes as well).
- Although not spelled out in the story, cultural attitudes regarding normative female development (the "princess" ideal) and ideal female body form (more slender than average) can damage girls' self-esteem, contribute to peer teasing and bullying, and skew parental expectations of girls in unhealthy ways.
- Secure attachment requires not only a stable home (which Dawn obtained at adoption) but also parental acceptance of the child "warts and all"; acceptance that is conditional upon fulfilling certain parental wishes usually does not result in a secure relationship.
- Emotional eating, self-induced vomiting, nonlethal self-injury (which can release endorphins and thus be emotionally calming), short-term sexual relationships, and even the repeated hospital visits all served to temporarily relieve Dawn's emotional distress and sense of emptiness, but none were healthy, reliable paths to emotional stability.
- Dawn's openness to joining a peer group (albeit an odd one), making friends, trying mindfulness practices, and engaging in therapy are all hopeful signs, as is her adoptive parents' recognition of their daughter's need for psychiatric care.

Finally, it is important to remember that this story could easily have had a different ending. Adolescents like Dawn may not always make deliberate suicide attempts, but their destructive attempts to regulate their emotions can have lethal consequences. Because of their repeated hospital visits for minor self-harm, emotionally unstable youth are sometimes not taken seriously. As the story illustrates, however, it is important not to miss potentially dangerous medical problems in this population. Given her unstable relationship history, it is also unclear whether or not Dawn will form a stable therapeutic relationship. Thus, her prognosis is still guarded.

CHAPTER 10

Communicating the Case Formulation and Its Treatment Implications

In this chapter, we consider how to best share the case formulation with the child, the family, and other professionals involved in the child's mental health care. Discussing the case formulation with children and families requires sensitivity and usually also includes some review of formulation-based treatment implications (discussed further in Chapter 11). Sharing the case formulation in written form can pose further challenges. Common difficulties with each of these aspects of sharing case formulations are illustrated with clinical examples.

Communication of the case formulation is shaped by the audience (child, family, mental health professional, or other party) and by the medium (oral vs. written communication). Usually, there is a discussion of the case formulation with the child and family before there is communication with other professionals (usually in the form of a written report), so the nature of this discussion will be considered first.

DISCUSSING THE CASE FORMULATION

Before You Talk to the Family

Before discussing the case formulation with the child and family, you need to think about how to best present it. Most practitioners find it helpful to take a few minutes alone to gather their thoughts before presenting their case formulation. When working on a mental health team, a discussion with colleagues that precedes the discussion with the family serves the same purpose.

Some important considerations include who should hear the case formulation together and who, separately; how much detail is helpful for each family member; what aspects should be emphasized in the discussion; and in what order various issues should be discussed.

Usually, it is best to present the case formulation to the parents and the child together so that everyone hears the same information presented in the same way. This approach minimizes misunderstandings and also reduces the temptation some practitioners face to side with either the child or the parents in the discussion. One cannot be too critical of any one person when everyone is in the same room, so the presentation becomes more objective, of necessity. In some cases, however, there is a rationale for presenting the case formulation separately to different family members.

Very young children may not understand the details of what is being discussed, so they often benefit from being provided a simpler version of the same information. Children who are not privy to certain family secrets should also be given an edited version of the case formulation. For example, recall the case of Jasmine in Chapter 7. Jasmine was a preschooler who was not aware of who her biological father was. In this situation, the practitioner elected to provide Jasmine with a separate, simple explanation of her difficulties that did not reveal her paternity. The sensitive issue of when to reveal the family's secret to Jasmine was further discussed with her parents during treatment, but it would have been premature to broach it at the time of assessment.

Teens may also benefit from some separate discussion of their difficulties, both to respect their autonomy and to avoid revealing to parents information that the teen is reluctant to share. Information pertaining to dangerous situations must always be shared to ensure safety, but often there is potentially embarrassing but harmless information that the teen prefers to keep private (e.g., having a "crush" on a particular peer, getting into trouble at school for minor, low-risk misbehavior). One option is to provide the teen a summary of the case formulation at the end of the individual interview, elicit his or her response, modify the case formulation accordingly, and then provide the revised version to parents and elicit their responses.

When presenting a case formulation, emphasizing the child and family's strengths is usually helpful, as many parents are discouraged or frustrated with the child by the time they seek a mental health assessment. "I'm glad we haven't missed the boat completely" or similar expressions of parental relief are common during a discussion of strengths. Building on strengths is also a useful intervention in most cases, so this emphasis leads nicely into a discussion of what strengths-based interventions would be helpful to the child. When parents are frustrated, discussing the child's strengths sometimes allows a shift in their perspective from seeing a "problem child" to "a child with strengths who happens to have a problem." Thus, the likelihood of the child being rejected or becoming a scapegoat for family problems is decreased.

The multifactorial nature of most mental health problems also deserves emphasis. Many parents are familiar with the idea of nature versus nurture and may assume that their child's difficulties will be attributed to one or the other. Therefore, I often start by talking about how mental health problems almost always emerge from an interaction between nature and nurture over the course of the child's life. These ideas lead nicely into a discussion of biological factors (i.e., "nature") and their interaction with children's familial, social, and cultural environment (i.e., "nurture") in relation to the child's psychological development at different ages. Before detailing these factors, I emphasize that no one factor explains all of the child's difficulties, but that the difficulties have emerged from a combination of different factors interacting over time.

When starting to discuss the factors, those for which there is substantial evidence and those that can be easily linked to helpful interventions deserve emphasis. For example, in the case of Abby (an anxious school-age girl with seizures discussed in Chapter 8), providing accurate information about how to best control her seizures reduced anxiety in both the child and her mother. Educational interventions are simple, fact based, and almost always helpful, so factors related to these interventions deserve emphasis. Similarly, in a child who is anxious about mathematics but clearly has limited mathematical ability (a factor that almost always contributes to this form of anxiety), one would emphasize the need to address mathematical ability, perhaps through tutoring in this subject. Factors that are less directly related to treatment or for which there is limited evidence should receive less emphasis and be stated tentatively. For example, in the rather complex case of Dawn in Chapter 9 it would be unfair to overemphasize the adoptive mother's unrealistic expectations of Dawn as a contributing factor, given Dawn's history of abuse, prenatal exposure to drugs, and numerous other risk factors. Of course, it would still be helpful for the adoptive mother to modify her expectations, but helping her do so would constitute one of many helpful interventions rather than becoming a major treatment focus.

To organize the presentation of the case formulation, it is often helpful to use the following order (or one quite similar to it):

- Restate the presenting problem in language that is understandable and acceptable to everyone in the room.
- If possible, link the presenting problem to a mental health diagnosis or treatable condition (e.g., negative, attention-seeking behavior is not a diagnosis but can certainly be treated with behavior modification).
- Talk about the multifactorial nature of mental health problems and the need to consider strengths as well as problems.
- Present risk and protective factors chronologically, as formulated, with more emphasis on those that are more relevant to intervention or less speculative and less emphasis on those that are less relevant to intervention or more speculative.
- Elicit the child and family's reactions to these ideas (see pp. 188–190).
- Link the case formulation to a proposed treatment plan (see pp. 190–191).
- Elicit the child and family's reactions to the proposed treatment plan (see pp. 191–192).
- Discuss documentation of the findings (including asking about any nonessential details the family does not want included in the report) and communication with other professionals involved in the child's mental health care.

The Nature of the Discussion

Sometimes practitioners assume that the case formulation is communicated to children and parents briefly at the end of an assessment and is presented as a complete, unalterable package. Nothing could be further from the truth.

It is important to take time to discuss the formulation with the child and family and to ensure that all participants are engaged in the discussion. Presenting a quick summary when there is little time for discussion is usually not in the child's best interest, as this approach may result in misunderstandings or alienation of the child and family. Sharing thoughts about the factors contributing to the child's difficulties often prompts children or parents to provide additional information that supports or refutes these ideas, resulting in a more accurate case formulation. For example, I once saw a child with severe separation anxiety whose father had suffered from a serious illness 3 years prior to the assessment, and I cited this illness as a possible contributing factor to the child's anxiety. In response, the father revealed that he had recently suffered a recurrence of his illness but had not yet shared this information with the child. Clearly, the recurrence was relevant to the child's current anxiety symptoms.

In addition to eliciting new information, discussing the case formulation sometimes reveals a "hidden agenda" that the family was hoping to address and that will need to be dealt with before planning treatment. For example, I once saw a recently separated couple in which the mother was hoping that my case formulation would attribute her child's depression entirely to her husband's recent departure, resulting in the husband feeling obligated to return "for the sake of the child." When I shared my impression that constitutional factors and parental conflict were contributing to the child's depression as well, she was clearly upset and unimpressed. Taking the time to address her reaction, however, allowed me to empathically explore her concerns about the recent dissolution of her marriage and then return to a discussion of what treatment might benefit her child. Consistent with this approach, some authors see the discussion of the case formulation as a first step in treatment planning (Persons, 2008, pp. 158–162). They suggest routinely emphasizing the parts of the formulation most relevant to treatment when communicating the case formulation to clients.

To ensure child and family engagement in the discussion, it is important to ask questions about their understanding of the case formulation and to discuss their agreement or disagreement with it. Such questions might include:

- "How does that sound to you?"
- "Do you have questions about what I just described?"
- "Does that make sense, or do you disagree with some of it?"
- "Are these ideas consistent with your understanding of the problem?"
- "Is there anything I've missed that would be important in understanding this problem?"
- "Would you be willing to proceed like this?" (if some aspects of treatment have been discussed).

Depending on the responses to these questions, the practitioner may then choose to explore certain issues further, resulting in a more complete and more accurate case formulation.

In addition, it is sometimes useful to ask children or parents to summarize the main issues in their own words, which allows the practitioner to check for misunderstandings about the case formulation. For example, despite my best efforts to emphasize the multifactorial nature of mental health problems, one or more family members may still summarize the main issues by blaming themselves or others. Thus, "Your child has always had a somewhat anxious temperament, but the anxiety was clearly exacerbated by the bullying at school last year" may be interpreted as "No matter how much she was bullied, it's my fault because everyone in my family is anxious, so I gave her the anxiety genes." It is important to address this misinterpretation, because self-blaming parents are often pessimistic about their ability to be helpful to the child.

During the discussion, it is helpful to observe body language as well as listening to participants' responses. For example, sometimes clients will offer verbal agreement with the case formulation but look very uncomfortable. It is important to gently confront this discomfort by saying "You look concerned about what I've just said. Is there something about it that doesn't seem quite right?" Alternatively, some clients offer verbal agreement but indicate with a wink or other dismissive expression that they do not feel the need to take the practitioner's comments seriously, or that they think the practitioner is saying certain things for the benefit of another family member. Such gestures are more difficult to confront directly and so often merit a separate interview with the family member who makes them.

In addition to disagreeing with the practitioner, family members can also dispute the formulation among themselves. For example, teenagers may believe their problems are their parents' fault or may believe that they have no problems at all. Parents of adolescents may have the opposite biases. Emphasizing the circularity of parent–teen interactions (as described in Chapter 9) is often helpful so that both sides can focus on changing a pattern of interaction rather than blaming each other.

The views of younger children may also differ from their parents' perspectives. In part, this is due to cognitive immaturity. For example, a young child may assume that she is upset because of a fight with a friend yesterday but may not be able to understand the reasons why the friend's behavior provoked anger. By contrast, the child's parent may be able to see how unfavorable comparisons with a very accomplished sibling made the child prone to anger toward peers, especially when the peers are particularly successful. Acknowledging the validity of both perspectives often allows the practitioner to work within both frames of reference as needed.

Disagreements between parents about the child's difficulties are also common, even when the marital relationship is otherwise good. For example, it is not unusual for one parent to sympathize with the child's problems and vulnerabilities, while the other parent sees the child as spoiled or manipulative. In this case, it is important to emphasize the need for parents to reach a common "middle ground" so they can work together effectively in managing the child's behavior. Addressing this need may become an important aspect of the child's treatment.

As in client–practitioner disagreements, it is important to attend to body language suggesting that family members disagree and gently confront such issues if possible. For example, sometimes parents (who often request mental health assessment on behalf of the child) listen attentively to the practitioner's impressions while their child or teen plays a game on a handheld electronic device. My usual response to this situation is to emphasize that the child or teen is an important participant in the discussion and to offer to discuss the case formulation with him or her separately from the parents if desired. Most youth elect to put down the electronic device at this point, though some elect to talk separately. The youth's choice and the parents' reaction to it often provide additional information about family dynamics. Normalizing some disagreement among family members is also often helpful so that families do not fear being labeled "dysfunctional" for their differences of opinion.

Moving toward a Treatment Plan

As mentioned, discussion of the case formulation is often an important prelude to treatment. This is true whether the practitioner intends to provide that treatment or the practitioner is serving as a mental health consultant to others who will provide the treatment. The more clearly children and families understand the proposed treatment plan and its rationale, the more likely they are to follow through on it. Thus, an important function of communicating the case formulation is to provide a clear rationale for the treatment proposed.

Ideally, addressing the various risk factors and strengthening the various protective factors identified in the case formulation should provide an outline of the treatment plan. Realistically, it may not be possible to address all factors (e.g., some constitutional factors may be difficult to modify), some interventions may not be readily available (e.g., some specialized psychotherapies such as CBT or dialectical behavioral therapy are not available in all communities), and some thought may be needed about the relationship between interventions suggested by the case formulation and evidence-based care (discussed further in Chapter 11), but the case formulation nevertheless provides a good starting point for treatment planning. Discussion of the treatment plan should include not only the nature of the interventions proposed but also the goals of each treatment, the roles of the participants in each treatment (youth, parents, therapist, etc.), the time frame of each treatment, the expected rate of progress with each treatment, and the relationships among treatments in the plan. For example, it is important to indicate whether proposed treatments will happen concurrently or in sequence, and whether or not there will be a reassessment or further care when the treatment(s) end (Manassis, 2009a, pp. 53–67).

It is important to invite questions about the treatment plan and the rationale for it. Asking the youth and parents to summarize their understanding of the proposed plan and their own roles in it is often a useful way to avoid misunderstandings. For example, I might say to parents something like "We will work together to find better ways of managing your child's behavior and to support his [or her] emerging ability to recognize and regulate feelings. Consistent, weekly meetings are going to be essential to making progress." The parents' version, however, might be something like "We will bring our child to you weekly unless it interferes with baseball practice. You will teach him [or her] coping skills." In this case, both the need for greater parental involvement in treatment and the need to prioritize treatment ahead of other extracurricular activities must be discussed further.

It is not always possible to reach a clear understanding and agreement to all aspects of the treatment plan in a single session. If certain aspects still seem unclear or controversial, book a session for further discussion if possible. Sometimes providing a brief consultation does not allow for such a further session. In this case, spell out clearly to the consultee what aspects of the plan require further discussion with the child or family before being implemented. If another session is possible, start it by explaining the rationale for treatment again, relating it to the case formulation previously presented (i.e., do not assume children and parents remember what was presented in the previous session in detail). Then elicit further child and family reactions to the treatment plan.

Sometimes this process may result in a discussion of the pros and cons of certain treatment options. This weighing of pros and cons is particularly common when recommending psychiatric medications for children and youth. In each case, the risks of providing—or not providing—medication need to be weighed against the potential benefits of providing—or not providing—medication. For example, in the case of children who suffer significant impairment from their symptoms, the risks of medication may include certain side effects, but the risks of not providing medication may include deterioration in functioning at school or socially. The benefits of medication may include the alleviation of symptoms, possibly improved functioning, and possibly greater amenability to other interventions (e.g., psychotherapy), but the benefits of not providing medication include avoiding medication-related side effects. The same risk–benefit analysis should ideally be done for psychotherapeutic interventions as well as medical ones to ensure that participants provide informed consent for all treatments (Persons, 2008, pp. 158–162). An approach to persistent disagreements about treatment is described further in Chapter 11.

PRESENTING THE CASE FORMULATION IN WRITTEN FORM

When writing up the case formulation, a simple guideline is "write for your audience." When writing for families use lay language, when writing for physicians use medical terms, and when addressing psychologists or other practitioners, use mental health terminology. Unfortunately, in complex cases all of these audiences may need a written version of the case formulation. Does this imply writing a version for each audience? Not necessarily. A more efficient approach is to write one report and attempt to make it suitable for all audiences.

Using a single report has the additional advantage of reducing misinterpretations of the case formulation that can result when slightly different language is used in different reports. For example, the impact of a possible learning disability on a school-age girl's mental health could be described in lay language as "Jenny has had trouble reading for years, so now she expects that anything she reads will be difficult even before she looks at it. She's not confident at all about her school-work." When writing for a medical professional, one might say, "Jenny's possible dyslexia is impacting her confidence at school." When writing for a psychologist, one might say, "As a result of prolonged reading dif-ficulty, Jenny now responds to reading materials with learned helpless-ness, reducing her confidence regarding academic work." In this case, the communication for physicians is quick and diagnostically focused, as their goal is to refer the child to the most appropriate mental health professional for further assessment and treatment. However, the lack of detail in this description might result in the mistaken impression that Jenny has already been diagnosed as dyslexic, even though she is still in need of academic assessment. The more detailed communication for psychologists, on the other hand, uses the term "learned helpless-ness," which might be confusing for a layperson. A generic description suitable for all audiences might be "As a result of prolonged reading problems, Jenny lacks confidence with schoolwork and is reluctant to attempt it."

There is some debate about the necessity of providing families with a written report, and whether or not the case formulation report sent to the family should be the same one sent to mental health professionals involved in the child's care. Some practitioners feel inhibited knowing that parents will read the report, a factor that might result in overly cau-tious, vague, or tentative wording. Others feel that writing with parents in mind minimizes pejorative language, ensures honesty about one's degree of certainty or uncertainty regarding the role of various factors in the child's presentation, and keeps everyone literally "on the same page" with respect to treatment planning. In the absence of a written report, families may selectively remember those parts of the case for-mulation they found reassuring and ignore other aspects, sometimes complicating treatment planning. For example, parents who hope to address their child's problems with psychotherapy may remember that psychotherapy was recommended but forget that a psychoeducational assessment for learning disabilities (which they hope their child does not have) was also deemed essential.

On balance, I believe there are more advantages to providing fami-lies and professionals the same report than not doing so. When writing that report, however, attention to certain details is required. The report writer should pay particular attention to the following:

• Avoid psychological or medical jargon. If a psychological or medical term must be used (e.g., reporting a specific diagnosis), the term should be described briefly in brackets when first used in the report. For example, "This child appears to have generalized anxiety disorder (tendency to worry excessively)."

• Avoid statements that might be offensive to the child or the parents. For example, rather than saying "This child seems developmentally delayed" in a situation in which the parents are not prepared to accept this conclusion and no formal intelligence test has been done, one might say "Clarification of this child's intellectual strengths and weaknesses is needed" and recommend further testing. Similarly, rather than saying "This mother seems to be undermining attempts to return the child to school," one might say "Aspects of the parent–child interaction may be contributing to school avoidance and merit further exploration." Pejorative statements almost always relate to factors that are not completely certain and therefore merit further investigation, so it is usually best to reword them and encourage such investigation.

• As previously discussed, emphasize the multifactorial origins of the problem, the child's and family's strengths, factors that can be readily linked to interventions, and factors that are certainly contributing to the problem(s) rather than those that are speculative.

• Avoid including information or ideas that have not been communicated to the family orally. If you have an additional idea after the family leaves the office, include it only if it is crucial to the child's well-being, and indicate in the report that this point was not discussed with the family. The family should find the report a helpful reminder of what was discussed, not a source of new information or new, surprising ideas.

• Provide your contact information so that anyone who has questions about the report can clarify them. This practice is particularly important when families and practitioners have very different perspectives on the child's problems, resulting in a report that has undergone significant editing to minimize the chances of offending anyone. In this case, a conference call among mental health providers can also be helpful in coordinating optimal care for the child.

• Indicate with "cc" who has received copies of the report. Families need to be reassured that their child's information has only been sent to professionals they have authorized to view it, and professionals need to be aware that families have received the report and it has been worded accordingly.

- Regardless of how tentative the case formulation may sound, ensure that your recommendations are clear, concise, and practical. Provide only as many recommendations as can be reasonably implemented. For example, in a case as complex as Dawn's (Chapter 9) one could probably generate a long list of possible interventions, but this would not be very useful. Reports with four to six clear recommendations (generally, one or two for parents, one or two for the child, one or two for referring professional or school) are more likely to result in a realistic treatment plan than those with dozens of nonspecific suggestions with no clear indication of who is to implement them and in what order they are to be pursued. Recommendations should address the key contributing factors to the child's problems that can be dealt with at any one time. A plan for future interventions can be outlined if desired, but one must recognize that such a plan is dependent on the child's response to the initial four to six interventions.

- Keep the report brief, if possible. Most busy professionals do not read more than the final page of any report, so this page should contain (at minimum) the key points of the case formulation, the main treatment recommendations, and your contact information.

To practice revising reports to make them informative and palatable to all readers, see if you can spot the difficulties in the following brief case formulation report. Then try and rewrite it so it could be sent to both the family and the referring professional with little risk of adverse responses. One possible revision of this report is provided at the end of this chapter (p. 197)

> "George is an 8-year-old boy, the youngest of three children, who presents with symptoms of oppositional defiant disorder. His mother's anxiety problems and George's position as the "baby" of the family have resulted in coddling and a lack of consistent behavioral limits. His father appears unable to support his wife in managing George's behavior, probably because of the amount of time he spends at the local bar. At school, George's motivation is low, as he would probably rather be at home manipulating his mother. He also has a December birthday, and so is the youngest in his class. He also doesn't seem that bright, although he does have some friends. George's parents would benefit from a Webster-Stratton parenting program, some marital counseling, AA for the father, and CBT for the mother."

In addition to writing reports carefully, it is important to have a clear understanding with families about who will see the report. Parents and (in the case of older adolescents) the youth must consent to the disclosure of their personal information to anyone outside the family. I usually tell families that I will send the report to them and to their referring professional (often a family doctor or pediatrician) unless they indicate otherwise. If there is another mental health professional likely to be involved in the child's treatment, I ask their permission to send the report to that person as well.

Some parents would like to share mental health information with the child's school. I usually do not suggest sending the full report to the school, however, as there is still considerable stigma about mental health issues in some schools. Also, there may be details about the family psychiatric history or other personal information that is relevant to the case formulation but not necessarily important for the school to know, and that could be potentially embarrassing to the family if disclosed. I often suggest either (1) sending a short excerpt from the report, containing the child's diagnosis(es), any relevant recommendations, and my contact information, to the school; or (2) having the parents read the full report and decide for themselves what aspects to share with the school. When in doubt, the second option usually ensures the best protection of private information.

A more difficult situation can arise if parents disagree strongly with the case formulation and do not wish to share the report. In some jurisdictions (including my own) the referring professional is still considered part of the child's circle of care and is therefore entitled to the report. In other jurisdictions, however, this is not the case. Usually, it is prudent for the practitioner to respect the family's wishes about not sharing the report. However, I usually try to elicit the family's agreement to at least inform the referring professional that (1) a mental health assessment of the child took place, and (2) I am not sharing the findings at the family's request. These two facts are often very informative to the referring professional and helpful to his or her further planning for the child's care. Unfortunately, the assessing practitioner cannot help the child with his or her mental health problems in this situation. There may still be some value, however, in the child hearing the discussion of the case formulation with the family. In this discussion, the practitioner (at minimum) demonstrates to the child that the parental worldview is not the only one and allows for the possibility that he or she may want to pursue mental health care in the future.

One possible revision of the case formulation report for George:

"George is an 8-year-old boy, the youngest of three children, who presents with symptoms of oppositional defiant disorder (a tendency to argue and refuse to obey the rules more than most boys his age). George was born the youngest of three children and has also consistently been the youngest in his class because he has a December birthday. His position as the youngest both at home and at school may contribute to George's perception of himself as immature and thus limit his motivation to engage in mature, task-oriented behavior. At school, his youth also places him at a disadvantage academically. A family history of anxiety in George's mother and possible substance abuse in his father may also make George vulnerable to poor emotional control, contributing to his acting-out behavior. Parental difficulty in managing his behavior consistently may be further exacerbating George's oppositional tendencies. Despite his behavioral and academic difficulties, George is well liked and has a number of friends. His social abilities are therefore a clear area of strength. George's parents also showed a willingness to acknowledge and address their own mental health concerns, and to work together in the best interest of their son. They would benefit from an evidence-based parenting program (e.g., the Webster-Stratton program) to better manage George and were also encouraged to ask their family doctor about resources to address their own respective mental health concerns. Given George's academic struggles, further clarification of his intellectual strengths and weaknesses is also needed."

CHAPTER 11

Using the Formulation
to Inform the Treatment Plan

After completing and communicating the case formulation, clinicians usually have a good (though not necessarily complete) understanding of children's mental health difficulties. Using that understanding to guide treatment, however, may require some further thought.

It is often helpful to think about treatment planning as a problem-solving process. That is, one begins by generating a list of possible interventions, then selects those interventions that appear feasible and are acceptable to the child and family, and then organizes selected interventions into a plan that can be implemented. One then ensures that all people involved in implementation agree on their respective roles and that there is a time to follow up with the child and family to review progress. The case formulation and the treatment plan may be revised on the basis of this progress review.

This chapter describes how to generate lists of interventions, select interventions, and organize a treatment plan. Case examples are used to illustrate these steps. Revision of the case formulation and treatment plan is described further in Chapter 12.

LISTING POSSIBLE INTERVENTIONS

As detailed in Chapter 1, it is important to consider both research evidence regarding treatments for certain child psychiatric diagnoses and an understanding of the child's difficulties drawn from the case formulation when considering possible interventions. Interventions suggested by the case formulation are usually complementary to those suggested by research evidence, rather than competing with them. For example, an adolescent with social anxiety may be referred to a cognitive-behavioral therapist on the basis of research evidence for this treatment of anxiety disorders. When exploring other risk factors for poor mental health as part of case formulation, however, a practitioner may discover a low level of physical activity in the teen. Therefore, the practitioner may recommend an enjoyable exercise program that includes peers, even though there is limited evidence that exercise reduces social anxiety.

Sometimes, the case formulation suggests modification of evidence-based treatment. For example, recall Malcolm's dilemma in Chapter 1. Although research evidence suggests that CBT for anxiety disorders is equally effective whether provided in group or individual format, there is little research data on providing this therapy to children like Malcolm who also have ADHD. A case formulation approach would have suggested individual treatment based on Malcolm's past learning difficulties in group situations.

Rarely does the case formulation guide practitioners away from evidence-based treatment. This situation might occur if the presenting diagnosis is masking a different underlying problem. For example, some children present with ADHD but have a history of significant trauma that is contributing to this presentation. In this case, the case formulation would suggest prioritizing psychotherapy to address the trauma, rather than medical treatment of the ADHD. It is unusual, however, for interventions based on case formulation to be inconsistent with evidence-based treatment.

Therefore, it is usually helpful to list and consider interventions tailored to both the child's psychiatric diagnosis and the risk and protective factors in the child's formulation. Figure 11.1 provides a sample grid for doing so. Once the list of interventions is complete, one can indicate on the grid which ones are likely to be feasible and acceptable to the child and family. Those that are both feasible and acceptable form the basis of the treatment plan. However, interventions that target what are thought to be the main factors contributing to the child's problem must be prioritized. Sometimes numerous possible interventions are suggested by the case formulation, and it is not realistic to implement them all at once. This issue is discussed further in the section below on organizing and implementing a treatment plan.

To illustrate how to use Figure 11.1 when planning treatment, let's

Intervention Type	Specific Intervention	Feasible?	Acceptable?	Priority?
Based on the child's diagnosis				
Based on risk factors				
Based on protective factors				

FIGURE 11.1. Grid of possible interventions.

examine some possible lists of interventions for children of different ages. One example is provided for each age group in Figures 11.2, 11.3, and 11.4. In Figure 11.2 we revisit Jasmine from Chapter 7, a preschooler who threatens her brother but has a complex family history of parental trauma and immigration that undoubtedly affected her psychological development. Figure 11.3 focuses on Malcolm from Chapter 1, a school-age boy who struggles with both anxiety and inattention as his parents are caught up in a bitter separation and divorce. Dawn from Chapter 9, a troubled teen with an eating disorder, self-harm behavior, and a

Intervention Type	Specific Intervention	Feasible?	Acceptable?	Priority?
Based on the child's diagnosis	• *No diagnosis was given in this case, though "oppositional defiant disorder" might be considered. If so, <u>parent training</u> in behavior management is indicated.*	Yes, for mother; no for father	Yes	
Based on risk factors	• *Treat mother's probable PTSD and traumatic grief*	Yes	Yes	Yes
	• *<u>Individual</u> treatment for Jasmine to improve self-regulation*	Yes	Yes	
	• *Psychological intervention focusing on mother and child (e.g., child–parent psychotherapy) or father and child*	Yes for mother/ child; no for father/ child	Yes	Yes (mother/ child)
	• *Positive peer experiences for Jasmine where she is not in a competitive or controlling role*	Yes	Yes	Yes
Based on protective factors	• *Psychoeducation of psychologically minded parents regarding Jasmine's difficulties so they can support her better*	Yes	Yes	Yes
	• *Community support (e.g., relief from some household chores for mother; occasional babysitting of infant brother) to allow time for mother and daughter to participate in treatment and spend time together*	Yes	Yes	Yes

FIGURE 11.2. Possible interventions for a preschooler (Jasmine).

history of sexual abuse, is the focus of Figure 11.4. Each case will be discussed further later in the chapter.

Note that only the interventions which are *not* already suggested by the child's diagnosis are indicated in the "based on risk factors" and "based on protective factors" categories. In other words, interventions based on case formulation often overlap with those based on diagnosis. Also, the interventions listed are limited to those commonly available

Intervention Type	Specific Intervention	Feasible?	Acceptable?	Priority?
Based on the child's diagnosis	• Stimulant medication for ADHD	Yes	No	
	• CBT for anxiety (any format)	Only if individual	Yes	
	• Parent behavior management training	Yes	Unlikely	
Based on risk factors	• Individual CBT	Possibly	Yes	Yes
	• Marital counseling for parents and/or mediation of parental divorce	Yes	Possibly	Yes
	• Case conference between family, mental health provider, and school personnel	Yes	Unlikely	
	• School modifications to improve attention (e.g., preferential seating, redirection)	Yes	Yes	Yes
Based on protective factors	• After-school activity involving peers and (ideally) sympathetic teacher	Yes	Yes	Yes
	• Support group for children of families undergoing divorce	Yes	Possibly	

FIGURE 11.3. Possible interventions for a school-age child (Malcolm).

in my practice. You may have access to additional ones in your community. To practice treatment planning, try listing possible interventions for the remaining case examples from previous chapters (Max, Abby, Serena, Raj, and Paul) according to your knowledge of evidence-based treatments and of the respective case formulations.

SELECTING INTERVENTIONS

As already stated and as the figures suggest, one wants to select for implementation those interventions that appear both feasible and acceptable to the child and family. By anticipating problems with

Intervention Type	Specific Intervention	Feasible?	Acceptable?	Priority?
Based on the child's diagnosis	• Medical treatment of cardiac and metabolic problems	Yes	Yes	Yes
	• Family therapy focused on healthy eating behaviors and appropriate autonomy to address eating disorder	Yes	Yes	Yes
	• Dialectical behavior therapy to improve emotion regulation and reduce self-harm	Yes	Yes, if female therapist	Yes
Based on risk factors	• Psychoeducational assessment to optimize learning	Yes	Yes	
	• Vocational assessment to set appropriate long-term goals	Yes	Yes	
	• Nutritional counseling	Yes	Yes	
	• Including attachment focus in family therapy	Yes	Yes	Yes
	• Including identity focus in individual therapy	Yes	Yes	Yes
	• Utilizing female therapists	Yes	Yes	Yes
Based on protective factors	• Peer group activity to foster healthy friendships and social connection	Yes	Yes	
	• Volunteer work in the community	Yes	Possibly	

FIGURE 11.4. Possible interventions for an adolescent (Dawn).

certain interventions, one can often prevent premature termination or treatment failure.

In some cases, the feasibility or lack of feasibility of an intervention seems obvious. For example, certain treatments may not be available in the client's community or may only be available at a cost the client's family cannot afford. In my own jurisdiction, specialized psychotherapies such as CBT or dialectical behavioral therapy fall into this category for clients living outside major urban centers. Interventions that require parents to take extensive time off work may also not be feasible in some families. For example, child–parent psychotherapy involving father and child would not be feasible in Jasmine's case because of the need for Jasmine's father to support his family financially. In short, a variety of logistical issues can prevent implementation of certain interventions.

In other cases, however, obstacles to implementation may have to be inferred from information about past treatment attempts and about child, family, and therapist characteristics. Information regarding previous interventions, successful or unsuccessful, is almost always useful in treatment planning. For example, I sometimes see parents of adolescents who report that their son or daughter did not feel comfortable "opening up" to three or more previous therapists, but then insist they want psychotherapy for the youngster. I usually respond by asking the family what has changed about the adolescent since the last attempted therapy. If neither the parents nor the adolescent can answer this question, I usually express skepticism about the chances of successful individual therapy. One or two failed attempts at therapy could be due to poor "fit" between therapist and client, but more than two usually suggests some form of resistance to the process in the client. In younger children, a common complaint about past therapy is "My child enjoyed going, but did not apply anything he/she learned in real life." In this case, I usually suggest a short series of sessions to review what was learned and then use concrete reminders and parental support to help transfer skills learned in the office to daily life. This practice acknowledges that there was some value to the previous therapy, reducing discouragement about the result, and avoids excessive repetition of material learned, which children often find boring.

Characteristics of the child, family, and therapist can also determine whether or not a particular intervention is feasible. Severe externalizing behavior in the child, for example, is disruptive to most individual therapies that target internalizing symptoms such as anxiety or depression. Children who act out when distressed may also lack the motivation to learn how to manage their feelings in other ways. Cognitive limitations in the child may be problematic in certain therapies (e.g., CBT). Most psychotherapies also require that families are organized enough to bring their children to appointments consistently and that parents play at least a small part in facilitating the child's progress. Parents who feel that the therapist must "fix" the child's problems with no participation on their part are often disappointed. The fit between therapist and child or therapist and family can also affect feasibility. For example, some families may be uncomfortable with therapists who are unfamiliar with their culture, and some children may be uncomfortable with therapists who remind them of negative past experiences (the latter is termed "transference" in psychoanalytic therapies). Dawn in Chapter 9, for example, reacted very negatively to male therapists, likely because their gender reminded her of past experiences of sexual abuse. Experienced therapists are also aware of their own strengths and weaknesses with respect to different types of clients. For example, some therapists struggle with children who are very quiet and require a patient, sensitive approach in order to engage in therapy, while others struggle more with those who are talkative and need frequent redirection.

The need to select interventions that are acceptable to the child and family reminds us that treatment planning must always involve a discussion with clients and their parents, which often includes some negotiation. Reasons that treatments may not be considered acceptable include lifestyle concerns, culturally based treatment preferences or prohibitions, fear of certain treatments due to misinformation, and low motivation to participate in the treatment plan proposed. For example, interference with school or important after-school activities may hamper treatment in some cases. Providing explanatory notes for teachers and scheduling treatment sessions at the beginning or end of the workday can minimize effects on school attendance and performance. On the other hand, when there is conflict between treatment times and after-school activities, families may need to prioritize one or the other. If the child's difficulties are substantial, suspending an after-school activity for a few months in order to pursue treatment is usually considered acceptable.

Medical treatments are sometimes declined owing to cultural prohibitions or misinformation. Cultural prohibitions are worth exploring in detail, with a cultural interpreter if necessary, to ensure that families have accurate information and are not interpreting cultural requirements in an overly stringent manner. For example, in some countries the color of a medication may be significant, portending good luck, bad luck, or even death. Misinformation is often more challenging to address, as this may require family education about the quality of various types and sources of information. It is surprising, for example, how many well-educated parents assume that anecdotal information they read on a website has the same credibility as a randomized controlled trial published in a peer-reviewed journal.

Motivation to pursue treatment may be generally low or may be affected by disagreements regarding the formulation or the specific treatment(s) proposed. Generally low motivation usually relates to failing to acknowledge there is a problem or not feeling ready to address the problem. Motivational interviewing techniques have been described to address these difficulties (Miller & Rollnick, 2013). Such techniques may need to be used with children, parents, or both depending on what is needed. For example, sometimes parents are motivated to pursue a particular treatment but the child is not, or vice versa. In younger children, motivated parents can often convince the child to participate in treatment for a few sessions, giving the therapist a chance to develop a therapeutic alliance with the child. In adolescents this is typically less successful, so motivational interviewing with the adolescent must be prioritized.

In some cases, however, motivation appears to be low because of unacknowledged disagreement with the formulation or the treatment plan. Some children and parents need more than one session to understand and "digest" the information presented to them at the end of an assessment. They may disagree with the treatment plan but not be able to articulate exactly why. At a subsequent visit, the reasons why certain interventions are not acceptable to them or not feasible may become clearer. Therefore, it is usually worthwhile booking an additional session for discussion when families do not appear eager to pursue treatment, particularly in complex cases.

If there is still substantial disagreement after this further session, however, the practitioner may need to "agree to disagree" with the family. Options at this point include referral to a colleague who might offer treatment that the family would consider more acceptable or a compromise that includes treatment elements agreeable to both sides. In the latter case, however, the practitioner must be careful to spell out the pros and cons of the modified treatment and the limits of that treatment, and state that he or she may elect to stop if there is no evidence of progress after a certain time. For example, I sometimes see children such as Malcolm (in Chapter 1) who have ADHD in addition to an anxiety disorder. Families are sometimes unwilling to consider medication for the ADHD until all psychotherapeutic options have been exhausted. After explaining to parents that children with unmedicated ADHD may have a suboptimal response to CBT for anxiety, I sometimes offer to see these children for a short series of sessions (usually three or four sessions) to determine their ability to benefit from therapy. I also explain to parents that the therapy is anxiety specific and therefore unlikely to affect ADHD symptoms. I then negotiate an agreement with the parents that if their child is too unfocused to retain any of the information from the initial three or four sessions then the issue of medication will be revisited, and further sessions will be contingent on the outcome of that discussion. Because it is unethical for a practitioner to provide treatment that is clearly not helpful, there is a need to limit the duration of interventions that may or may not succeed.

The interventions listed in the case examples in the figures can now each be examined for feasibility and acceptability. Given the high level of motivation in Jasmine's family (Figure 11.2), no interventions were deemed unacceptable, but (as mentioned earlier) interventions involving extensive participation by Jasmine's father were not feasible because of his work commitments.

Malcolm's case (Figure 11.3) is somewhat more complicated. Almost all interventions are feasible in this case, although CBT needs to be provided on an individual basis and will only succeed if Malcolm's inattention is not too severe. Acceptability of many interventions is uncertain, however, in this highly conflicted family. Malcolm's mother clearly will not consent to medication for her son, and will consent to CBT because she attributes his difficulties to anxiety. She is unlikely to agree to behavior management training as this is an ADHD-focused intervention, and her husband is unlikely to agree to it because he does not think his son has a mental health problem. The parents might be willing to consider mediation of their divorce, although it would be challenging given their degree of conflict. They also might agree to a support group for Malcolm, as most children find parental divorce stressful and attending a support group does not imply that Malcolm has any particular mental health problem. The case conference with the school is unlikely to succeed, given the perception of Malcolm's mother that the teacher is incompetent. However, Malcolm's parents would likely not object to minor school modifications to improve his attention and his participation in a healthy after-school activity.

Dawn (Figure 11.4) has multiple problems, and so multiple interventions could be considered. All are feasible and almost all are acceptable to Dawn and her adoptive parents, but they clearly cannot all begin at once. Prioritization of interventions is needed and will be discussed further in the next section. It will be important to include mainly or exclusively female therapists in Dawn's care, given her aversion to working with males owing to past sexual abuse. Also, although volunteer work is a great source of self-esteem for many teens and it is a requirement for high school graduation in some jurisdictions, Dawn may be too overwhelmed with her problems to consider it immediately.

ORGANIZING AND IMPLEMENTING A TREATMENT PLAN

Once interventions that are not feasible or not acceptable to the child or family have been eliminated, the remaining interventions must be organized and prioritized to form a treatment plan. In order to implement this plan, all participants must be in agreement and must work together in a coordinated fashion. Formation and implementation of a treatment plan will now be discussed.

Sometimes, the treatment plan is very simple and based on a single intervention. For example, a young child with a specific phobia of dogs must undergo desensitization to dogs through repeated exposure exercises, usually with parental support. Often, however, treatment plans include several interventions that must be organized and prioritized in order to ensure that they succeed and that the child and family are not overwhelmed with multiple concurrent interventions. Careful thought is needed to decide where to start and which issues to address at the same time. Detailed descriptions of this process are included in books by Manassis (2009a, pp. 35–51) and Persons (2008, pp. 150–156, 232–235).

Some considerations when prioritizing interventions include the following:

• *Start with life-threatening issues.* For example, when children or teens experience suicidal thoughts, consider hospitalization before implementing other interventions. Similarly, when the child's psychiatric problems are resulting in a life-threatening medical condition, treatment of the medical condition may need to be prioritized. This occurred in Dawn's case when her bulimia resulted in an irregular heartbeat.

• *Start with issues likely to threaten the therapeutic alliance.* With the therapeutic alliance as the cornerstone for any successful treatment, monitoring and maintaining the connection between the practitioner and the family is paramount. For example, when children and parents cannot agree on the nature of the problem, you'll need to provide further education and discussion before moving forward. Family secrets can also threaten the therapeutic alliance, as keeping information from a child or a parent can make the therapist seem untrustworthy. Such secrets include facts that the parents do not wish to disclose to the child (as in Jasmine's case, in which her parentage was kept secret) and facts that the child or teen does not wish to disclose to the parents (e.g., alcohol or substance abuse that the child or teen is trying to hide). Not all secrets need to be revealed immediately, but the value of transparency over secrecy usually merits discussion in relation to psychotherapy, family relationships, and the safety and well-being of family members.

• *Start with issues that are highly impairing.* For example, a child with obsessive–compulsive disorder who compromises the rest of his life by spending several hours per day engaged in compulsive rituals may need medication in addition to psychotherapy to limit these behaviors. Without such treatment, the child's ability to function at home, at school, and with peers would be severely compromised.

- *Start with issues that can be quickly or easily addressed.* Interventions that reduce unnecessary stress in the child's life can often be implemented quickly and relatively easily. Examples include providing adult supervision in situations where children are repeatedly teased or bullied, implementing a predictable schedule of parental visits in divorced families, and ensuring that schoolteachers avoid anxiety-provoking practices such as evaluating students using unexpected quizzes or humiliating students who provide incorrect answers.

- *Start with an issue that has a high likelihood of furthering treatment.* Many interventions make it easier for children and families to subsequently participate in psychotherapy. Children in foster care, for example, often need a stable, trusting relationship with a foster parent or other reliable adult for a period of time before they can learn to trust a therapist. Families who are impoverished may need transit tokens or other financial support in order to facilitate consistent attendance at appointments.

- *Start in an area in which the child or family is motivated to work hard.* For example, I sometimes see children who are severely impaired in one area but more motivated to begin working on another area. I once saw a young teen on the autism spectrum who was highly motivated to overcome test-taking fears because they interfered with school success and therefore threatened his goal of becoming a pilot. My assessment also revealed very poor social skills with peers, but the boy had no desire to address these. I elected to begin with the area he wanted to pursue, which resulted in academic improvement and eventual participation in a school science club where his social skills also improved. Parents, on the other hand, sometimes present with significant personal mental health issues but are motivated to start with treatment for their children. If the child is agreeable and the parent's issues are not immediately threatening to the child's well-being, it is sometimes wise to begin with child treatment in the hope of engaging the family in a positive therapeutic experience that facilitates eventual treatment for the parent.

- *Start by building strengths and supports before tackling problems.* Most strengths and protective factors noted in the case formulation can be enhanced by attending to them consistently. The ability to relate to peers, for example, is a key strength that can be developed further by enrolling the child in a regularly scheduled activity involving other children. Community support can often be enhanced by encouraging parents to tell their friends, church members, and other community contacts what kind of help they need. Jasmine's mother, for example, benefitted greatly from household help and babysitting so she could attend to her daughter's needs.

Given the fact that several of these considerations may apply, practitioners must also consider the question: What interventions can be started *concurrently*? These should be limited to a manageable few to avoid overwhelming clients. Practitioners must also consider, however, what effect treating one problem will have on other problems and what effect one intervention will have on another intervention. Thus, when deciding whether to start several interventions concurrently or offer them sequentially, one must bear in mind several possible outcomes. These can include the following:

• *Treating one problem will resolve or improve another.* For example, treating depression can result in improved friendships and improved school functioning; ameliorating family conflict can result in reduced anxiety in children.

• *Treating one problem will exacerbate another.* Fortunately, this outcome is not common, but it can occur in some cases. For example, some adolescents with both anxiety disorders and conduct problems can show exacerbations in their behavior when their anxiety is treated, probably because they have less fear of the consequences of their actions.

• *Treating one problem will not affect the others.* This possible outcome is important to discuss with parents, as they may hope that treating one of the child's problems will resolve others. For example, parents may think that treating a child's ADHD with medication will result in improved behavior and improved school performance, but this does not always occur. In this case, the treatment targets a cognitive process (inattention) that may contribute to behavioral and school problems, but these problems may also depend on additional factors such as motivation and interpersonal skills.

• *One intervention will facilitate another.* Some examples of this process have already been mentioned. They include using motivational interviewing to facilitate subsequent psychotherapy and using medication that improves cognition to increase a child's ability to benefit from CBT. Interventions that reduce family discord (e.g., marital therapy or family therapy) can also be used to facilitate subsequent psychotherapy for individual family members.

- *One intervention will interfere with another.* Fortunately, this outcome is not common, but it can occur. For example, some children with anxiety or depression can be so effectively treated with medication that they display few remaining symptoms. Although often considered a positive outcome, this result may prevent the child from participating effectively in psychotherapeutic treatment as it leaves the psychotherapist with little to work with. Without psychotherapy, the child is left vulnerable to a subsequent relapse if medication is discontinued. Some forms of psychotherapy can also conflict with each other. For example, children who are enrolled in both psychodynamic or play therapy and CBT at the same time may achieve limited benefit from both because they entail different therapeutic goals. The first aims to weaken defenses in order to uncover underlying psychological conflicts; the second aims to strengthen coping strategies (many of which are similar or identical to defenses) in order to improve day-to-day functioning.

- *Interventions will operate independently.* This outcome commonly occurs when interventions target the child's behavior in different environments. For example, educational strategies may improve a child's academic performance but have little or no impact on social or family functioning; family therapy may improve home life but not school performance or peer relations. Sometimes, however, apparently independent interventions can mutually enhance each other over time. Thus, both educational strategies and family therapy can positively affect the child's self-esteem, which may be generally advantageous for development in the long term.

A final consideration when implementing treatment plans is the need to consult and coordinate all participants involved. This process must include not only mental health providers but also the child, the family, school personnel, sometimes a peer or peer group (e.g., when children are struggling socially), and sometimes other adults who are important in the child's life (e.g., a coach or activity leader; a member of the extended family). Even very good treatment plans are sometimes undermined by skeptical schoolteachers, unsympathetic peers, or respected grandparents who were not consulted when the plan was developed. It is not always possible to coordinate a single meeting that includes all participants, but practitioners should have at least one conversation with each person involved. Obtain permission to speak to these people from parents, and from youth as well in the case of older children and teens. Then contact each person by telephone or invite him or her to a subsequent appointment.

Sometimes people who seem peripheral to the plan can provide valuable additional information that sheds new light on the case. In other instances, they might show how some interventions would be helpful or anticipate obstacles to ones already planned. Finally, sometimes it is simply important to have their blessing in order for treatment to succeed. Moreover, coordinating the work of multiple people involves not only gathering information and eliciting agreement to a plan. It also requires scheduling and organizational skills, ensuring that no participant is either left out or overburdened with tasks, anticipating potential problems with implementation, and building in periodic opportunities for feedback and "fine-tuning" of the plan.

Let's apply some of these ideas to the examples in the figures. You may want to apply the ideas to some of the other longer examples (Max, Abby, Serena, Raj, and Paul) for practice. In the final column of the figures (Priority), I indicate one possible set of interventions that could be started concurrently for each case.

For Jasmine, I would elect to start with psychological intervention focused on mother and child and individual treatment of her mother for PTSD, given that much of Jasmine's difficulty relates to her attachment history and (more remotely) to her mother's traumatic history. As these treatments will involve a considerable time commitment for Jasmine's mother, community support regarding household chores and babysitting is also important. Jasmine's father cannot participate in treatment to the same degree as his wife, given his work schedule, but psychoeducation regarding Jasmine's difficulties is a brief intervention that could be helpful to both parents. Finally, positive, noncompetitive peer experiences for Jasmine will provide her with some practice at socially appropriate interactions for a child of her age and will probably be more fun than additional psychotherapy for a preschooler. Behavior management training is a good general parenting intervention but would not be a priority in this case given the specific link between Jasmine's behavior and the attachment history.

For Malcolm, I would start with urging marital counseling or divorce mediation for his parents, as parental conflict is undoubtedly contributing to his symptoms. Further interventions are limited to those that are acceptable to both of his parents, which are few. Given parental preferences and Malcolm's inattention, I would offer individual (not group) CBT, with the understanding that the question of medication might have to be revisited, depending on Malcolm's response after three or four sessions. Malcolm's parents would likely agree to school modifications to improve attention and an after-school activity involving peers, which could improve (respectively) his school and social functioning. They would be unlikely to agree to a school-based case conference, given the mother's tendency to blame school personnel for Malcolm's difficulties. They would be unlikely to agree to stimulant medication, at least as an initial intervention, given their stated preferences regarding treatment. They would be unlikely to agree to parent behavior management training, a helpful intervention for externalizing problems including ADHD, as the mother thinks her son suffers exclusively from anxiety and the father thinks he has no mental health problems. A support group for children of families undergoing divorce might be helpful to Malcolm at some point, but I might defer it initially in favor of an after-school activity because (1) it would be more stigmatizing to Malcolm than an after-school activity; (2) Malcolm will be busy enough with his individual therapy and after-school activity; and (3) it might reduce the parents' motivation to attend mediation, as they would assume that their son's divorce-related difficulties had been addressed.

In Dawn's case, it is obvious that her medical problems are life-threatening and must be addressed immediately. Next, the diagnostically based interventions must be prioritized. Family therapy focused on healthy eating behaviors and appropriate autonomy, including attention to attachment issues, is an important evidence-based treatment for her eating disorder. Dialectical behavior therapy is an evidence-based treatment focused on emotion regulation and reducing self-harm, which Dawn could clearly benefit from. Given her highly compromised medical state, I am less concerned about overburdening Dawn with therapy (i.e., starting both family and individual therapy at the same time) than I might be in other cases. In both therapies, it would be helpful to utilize female therapists if possible given Dawn's history of sexual abuse and of rejecting male therapists. There would also be a need to address Dawn's identity issues at some point in individual therapy, given the discrepancy between how Dawn sees herself and how her parents see her and, perhaps, how some of her peers see her. She also may need some support around becoming comfortable with her sexual orientation. The other assessments and interventions in Figure 11.4 are all important but may need to be introduced into the treatment plan gradually to avoid overwhelming Dawn and her parents.

In all of these cases, it would be important to consult and coordinate with everyone involved in the treatment plan. As mentioned, this process would include gathering information from each participant and eliciting agreement to the plan, organizing a schedule for various interventions, ensuring that no participant is either left out or overburdened with tasks, anticipating potential problems with implementation, and building in periodic opportunities for feedback and "finetuning" of the plan.

CHAPTER 12

Formulation Challenges
and the Need
to Monitor Progress

When clinicians implement treatment plans based on a detailed formulation, they hope for smooth sailing. They may anticipate that treatment will be effective, that the child and family will adhere to it, and that the problems will gradually resolve. Unfortunately, this is usually the exception, not the rule. Revision of the formulation, the treatment plan, or both may be needed before some children improve. In other children, challenges occur earlier in the process of assessment and treatment. Practitioners may struggle to arrive at a coherent formulation in these cases. This chapter examines such formulation challenges as well as situations in which revision of the formulation or treatment plan is needed.

CHALLENGES IN CASE FORMULATION

When thinking about challenges in case formulation, using the analogy of a jigsaw puzzle can be helpful. When solving such a puzzle, problems can include missing pieces, too many pieces to organize, pieces that don't seem to fit, and (in some cases) more than one apparent solution to the puzzle. Let's apply each of these possibilities to dilemmas in case formulation.

Missing Pieces

When a child's symptoms are more severe than his or her risk factors would predict, or the child's presentation appears unusual, the practitioner may be missing one or more key pieces of information. Most commonly, the "missing piece" is either an undiagnosed medical condition or an unreported stress in the child's life. For example, certain types of seizures (termed petit mal or absence seizures) can result in inattention in a child with no prior history of ADHD symptoms. This possibility should be considered in children who present with "late-onset ADHD." Traumatic events in the child's life can result in a similar presentation. Children who suddenly appear to have anxiety disorders but have no prior history of anxious temperament may also be suffering the effects of trauma or of a medical problem. Thyroid problems, diabetes, or undisclosed substance abuse are common in these cases. Psychotic symptoms are rare in prepubertal children, so a thorough medical investigation for various illnesses (e.g., diseases of the brain or systemic lupus) is indicated if these symptoms occur. Knowing the typical and atypical presentations of children's mental health problems is important, as it allows practitioners to advocate for medical investigations when the presentation is atypical.

Too Many Pieces to Organize

Complex formulations in which many risk and protective factors appear to be at play can be difficult to complete. This difficulty is most commonly encountered when seeing adolescents who have experienced many years of mental health difficulties but can occur in younger children as well. Sometimes a single assessment visit does not allow the practitioner to ascertain the precise connections among all risk and protective factors, but common overarching themes can usually be found. Once an overarching theme has been used to anchor the formulation, detailed connections among risk and protective factors can be explored over time to gain a more complete understanding of the child or adolescent's psychological struggles.

Difficulty regulating strong emotions (also termed "poor affect regulation") is one overarching theme, illustrated in the formulations of Dawn (a young woman with an eating disorder and self-harm behavior described in Chapter 9) and Serena (a girl of 11 years with severe oppositionality described in Chapter 4 and discussed further in this chapter). Factors that are associated with affect regulation difficulties in children and adolescents are described in detail in Bradley (2003).

The struggle to form a stable and positive identity is another common theme in adolescent case formulation. For example, Paul (a young teen with behavioral problems and substance abuse described in Chapter 2) had a stable but negative identity as a troublemaker. Raj (a boy with chronic school avoidance described in Chapter 9), on the other hand, does not appear to have concerns about his identity but seems to acquiesce to his family's perception that he is vulnerable and fragile. In this sense, Raj's formulation could also be organized around a negative personal identity. Identity is often a good overarching theme in this age group because it is essentially a product of how adolescents have dealt with previous psychological challenges.

Pieces That Don't Seem to Fit

Sometimes an assessment yields apparently contradictory information about the child, or the child's behavior actually appears to be contradictory. Both issues can cause problems when trying to develop a coherent formulation. Contradictory information is often provided when various informants have different perceptions of the child. Parents and teachers, for instance, often perceive different behaviors in children. If the child is truly behaving differently in different environments, such inconsistent behavior constitutes useful information that can be readily incorporated into the formulation (e.g., child behaves worst at home, where he or she feels safe to do so, but is anxious and therefore well mannered at school). If the different reports are due to conflict among the informants, however, obtaining accurate information about the child can be more difficult. Sometimes this difficulty occurs with home versus school conflicts, but more commonly it occurs when couples are separated or divorced and highly conflicted. In extreme cases, one parent may report that the child has no problems and is merely being "coached" to display symptoms by his or her ex-spouse, and the other parent reports the child meeting criteria for multiple psychiatric disorders. In these cases, neither parent may be a reliable source of information. Therefore, it is usually best to find an objective observer outside the family (usually a teacher, physician, or other mental health professional) to obtain accurate observations of the child's behavior.

Children who clearly demonstrate contradictory behavior require a different approach. In these cases, I usually assume that there is a piece of information that would resolve the contradiction, but the child is not comfortable telling me about it on the first visit. If I am starting psychotherapy with the child, the information is usually disclosed during a subsequent visit once a trusting therapeutic relationship has been established. If I am offering a consultation, I usually alert the consultee to the contradiction and the need for further gentle exploration. Examples include children who display signs of posttraumatic stress but do not report trauma initially, children who display compulsions but deny obsessions initially (as these are often embarrassing), or children who are reluctant to reveal certain family circumstances that are affecting their progress. The latter situation occurred, for example, with a young girl I was treating for social anxiety. She initially appeared motivated to join the Girl Guides as part of her desensitization to social situations but quit this activity after a single meeting. After asking a number of anxiety-related questions, I finally asked about other problems she might have encountered at Girl Guides. In tears, she confessed that the Guide leader had told all the girls to bring bleach bottles for the craft activity the following week, and she could not do so. Her impoverished family could not afford to buy bleach for the craft and did not use it routinely because they did not own a washing machine.

More Than One Solution to the Puzzle

Sometimes there are multiple ways of connecting various risk and protective factors in a case formulation and all appear to make sense. In this situation, the practitioner is left wondering which set of connections constitutes the "correct" formulation. For example, is a child with multiple siblings who cries when his mother goes to a different floor of the house exhibiting separation anxiety or attention-seeking behavior? Could the behavior be due to both factors? If both factors can be easily addressed, then determining the most salient factor may not be crucial. In this case, for example, positively reinforcing the child (i.e., providing extra attention) for tolerating a few minutes away from his mother without crying (i.e., desensitizing to the separation) would address both factors.

In other situations, however, it may be more difficult to address all possible factors, so the practitioner must pick one to intervene with and determine how important it is to the case formulation depending on the result. For instance, a promising 12-year-old hockey player who has recently been sidelined with a concussion presents with increasingly severe angry outbursts. There are multiple possible explanations for this behavior. As he is entering adolescence, he may want more independence from his parents. If they are reluctant to allow this, he may become angry. Alternatively, his mild head injury (i.e., the concussion) may be resulting in difficulty regulating negative emotions. Alternatively, he may be experiencing learning problems at school because of his head injury, resulting in frustration and anger. Alternatively, this active, athletic boy may be having difficulty coping with his lack of activity postconcussion and be desperate to return to playing hockey. Some of these possibilities are more easily addressed than others, and all will require some time to sort out before a definitive formulation can be developed.

REVISING THE CASE FORMULATION

As we consider the need for revision, it is worth revisiting the definition of the case formulation provided in Chapter 1. The three main elements to recall are: 1) the case formulation as hypotheses about factors contributing to a person's emotional and behavioral problems; 2) the case formulation as a means of organizing complex and sometimes contradictory information about a person's difficulties; 3) the case formulation as a blueprint for guiding treatment (Eells, 2006, p. 4). The word "hypotheses" reminds us that the case formulation is always somewhat tentative. It is the best model for the patient's problems we can design at a given time, but it may need to be revised in future. Figure 1.1 illustrates this revision process. Here, the treatment outcome, child development, and new information or events are all shown impacting the explanatory model of the child's difficulties (i.e., the case formulation). Thus, reasons for revision of the case formulation can include the following: new information about the child or family comes to light; developmental changes in the child affect the formulation; changes in the child's environment (i.e., events in the child's life) affect the formulation; or the child's response or lack of response to intervention affects the formulation. Revision may be needed almost immediately (e.g., if the family discloses additional information at the end of the initial assessment), after a short time (e.g., if the child discloses new information after a few sessions of psychotherapy), or after years (e.g., when the child and family return for further treatment or for a further consultation).

Regardless of the timing, it is important that practitioners not consider a need to change the formulation a professional failure. We all do the best we can with what we know at a given time, and (according to an old adage) hindsight is always 20/20. Of course, if one misses the same issue repeatedly, it is worth reflecting on this problem. Sometimes it is due to a personal blind spot (discussed at the end of the chapter). Sometimes practitioners are uncomfortable with one or more areas of inquiry and so neglect to ask certain questions. Questions pertaining to sexuality or sexual orientation, for example, are avoided by some practitioners. Others avoid questions about faith or spirituality. Awareness of the discomfort, however, allows practitioners to obtain guidance about how to best ask these questions. Then, with rehearsal and practice, they become easier to ask.

Revision Based on New Information, Developmental Changes, and Environmental Change

Let's examine new information, developmental changes, and changes in the child's environment in more detail before discussing treatment-related revisions. New information about the child that prompts revision can come from the child, the family, or research evidence. As mentioned, children often disclose additional information once they develop a trusting relationship with a therapist. Similarly, parents may disclose more sensitive information over time. Family dynamics may also become more apparent over time. This occurs because most families try to "put their best foot forward" at the initial assessment, which may prevent the practitioner from perceiving family conflict or other relevant family problems. It is also difficult for most practitioners to attend carefully to family interactions during the initial assessment, when they are in the midst of gathering information from parents and children. Research evidence pertaining to the causes of certain mental health problems can also alter the formulation. For example, many child mental health problems that were attributed to faulty parenting in the past are now seen as having biological antecedents, at least in part. Changes in diagnostic nomenclature can also influence the formulation. For instance, the change from the categorical diagnoses "Asperger's disorder" and "autism" (in DSM-IV) to the dimensional construct "autism spectrum" (in DSM-5) may influence our ideas about children with these problems.

Developmental changes can result in new strengths in the child as well as new challenges or deficits in relation to peers. New strengths often emerge as children adapt to the school setting and gradually develop executive functions that help regulate emotions. For example, a child who is suspended from day care for repeatedly having tantrums in response to transitions may become better able to tolerate transitions over time. The child's concept of time improves, allowing him or her to plan for changes, the child's ability to understand what is socially acceptable or unacceptable improves, and the child develops language and other abilities to help regulate strong feelings. On the other hand, children with learning disabilities who have good social skills may do well in preschool but face increasing challenges as academic requirements increase in the elementary and high school years.

All children experience periodic changes in their environment. Moving to a new home, changing schools, having close friends move away, and coping with the death of a pet are some common environmental changes that most children experience. Environmental changes that alter the child's psychological development more dramatically, however, often relate to serious illness or loss in the nuclear family. These so-called "major life events" remind us of how precarious our North American life balance can be. Most families' plans are based on the assumption that there are two healthy, working parents with one or two relatively healthy children. Realists may consider the (unfortunately common) possibility of parental divorce at some point, but other events are almost never anticipated.

When a serious illness, death, or family separation occurs, it often begins a cascade of events that impacts multiple aspects of child development. Emotional responses to the separation or the loss or illness of a family member represent only one aspect of these impacts. There are some excellent resources regarding children's responses to such events—for example, Grollman's (2011) book on talking to children about bereavement; Block, Kemp, Smith, and Segal's (2012) book on children's responses to divorce; and McCue's (1996) book on helping children cope with a parent's serious illness.

In addition to their emotional impact, however, these events alter children's and families' lifestyles and familiar routines irrevocably. Extensive medical appointments and medical procedures, or extensive legal appointments and legal procedures in the case of divorce or of settling an estate, add to the family burden by consuming time, energy, and financial resources. Eventually, this burden may make it difficult for one or both parents to continue working. Loss of employment then adds to the emotional and financial strain. Attention to ill family members may leave other members feeling neglected, heightening family conflict and potentially influencing neglected members to seek comfort outside the family (e.g., affairs in the case of neglected spouses; unhealthy peer relationships in the case of neglected children). Increased financial strain may necessitate a move, a change of schools, or other changes in family plans. Parental health may suffer, as parents become both physically and mentally exhausted. Exhausted parents have difficulty attending to their children's emotional needs, resulting in further problems in their development. In summary, the "domino effects" resulting from loss, family separation, or serious illness in the family can make a previously sensible formulation of a child's difficulties seem almost meaningless.

Revision Based on Treatment Response

Baselines

Before revising the formulation in relation to treatment response, one must have a clear idea of how much or how little response to treatment occurred. Few mental health treatments are completely curative, so measuring the degree of treatment response is important. Usually, this task is done every few weeks or at least every couple of months. In Chapter 2, the use of questionnaires to determine a baseline of symptom severity was discussed. Observational baseline measures, however, may also be useful. Children, adolescents, and adults around them can often quantify the severity of problems when asked to think about specific situations. For example, when an adolescent is depressed, withdrawn, and lethargic, the adolescent or a parent may be able to quantify how long the morning routine takes from wakening until (hopefully) catching the bus to school. Alternatively, the amount of self-care the adolescent does without parental prompting, the amount of time he or she spends among family or friends, or the amount of schoolwork he or she is still able to complete could be quantified.

Besides providing the practitioner with information on the degree of treatment response, and thus confirming or disconfirming formulation-related hypotheses, baselines can serve additional functions. For some clients, the need to monitor symptoms helps build an awareness of those symptoms. For example, a child may initially deny feeling anxious but start noticing anxious feelings when asked to monitor the frequency of his or her early-morning stomachaches. By revealing small signs of progress, baselines can also provide encouragement to children or families who are becoming discouraged with apparent lack of treatment-related progress. On the other hand, when baselines reveal a true lack of progress or even deterioration, clients and therapists are prompted to search for impediments to treatment success or to consider alternative treatments.

Sometimes, relationships between two or more baseline measures can also be informative and helpful. For example, in the case of the depressed, lethargic teen just mentioned, completion of schoolwork and a self-report questionnaire on mood could both be monitored regularly. Over time, these reports might reveal a relationship between increased schoolwork completion and improved mood. Although such relationships are not necessarily causal, they can be encouraging for clients to see and thus have positive effects on motivation. On the other hand, if one problem present at a baseline resolves but another becomes worse or a totally new problem emerges, it may be worth seeking a common source for the problems. For example, a young child with oppositional behavior at home and no prior history of learning problems might show improved behavior but begin failing at school. In this case, it is possible that both problems elicit negative parental attention, and the child is not used to eliciting parental attention in positive ways so persists with engaging in problem behaviors of one sort or another. Monitoring changes from a baseline may allow the practitioner to become aware of this pattern and address it with the child and family.

Changing Course or Not

Once a change from a baseline is detected, the practitioner tries to relate this change to the case formulation and to adjust the treatment plan if needed. If the change is in the expected direction, the case formulation is not changed and the treatment continues. Very slow change, however, may indicate a need to address additional contributing factors found in the case formulation, a need to increase treatment intensity (e.g., having more frequent sessions), or a need to look for possible nonadherence or other impediments to successful treatment. If there is no change or there is deterioration, revision of the case formulation and treatment plan may be needed.

One must be careful, however, not to assume that positive change with treatment proves that the case formulation or the diagnosis is correct. Some treatments are generically helpful. That is, they result in improved behavior for all children and adolescents and don't necessarily imply any particular psychological process. For example, almost all children appear happier and better behaved when they are provided with consistent praise and positive reinforcement for their efforts. Therefore, a positive response to this form of behavior management does not imply that the child was previously suffering from depression, low self-esteem, a behavioral disorder, or any other type of psychological problem. Similarly, almost all children and adults show an improved ability to focus their attention when given stimulant medication. Therefore, a favorable response to stimulant medication does not prove that a child has ADHD.

Deterioration with treatment or lack of change after several months may indicate a need to revise the case formulation. The child and family should be carefully reevaluated to elicit additional information, ascertain whether the child is facing a new stress or has undergone a developmental change, and look for possible treatment nonadherence or other impediments to treatment success. These impediments might include problems in the therapeutic relationship (e.g., children or parent are unclear about what is expected of them in treatment or what to expect of the therapist; poor "fit" between child and therapist or family and therapist; therapist "blind spots"—described at the end of this chapter); unrealistic or overly ambitious treatment goals resulting in discouragement; a secret need or wish harbored by the child or family that the treatment is not addressing; or logistical problems preventing the child or family from attending sessions consistently and making the therapeutic work a priority.

Inviting discussion of these issues in a friendly way is important. Rather than assuming that children or families are nonadherent or resistant to change, for example, begin with a gentle query such as "I wonder what is getting in the way of your child's progress. Do you have any ideas?" or "I thought we would have solved at least one of these problems by now, but it seems we're stuck. Why do think that's happening?" If the response is a shoulder shrug, it may help to elicit feedback more directly by asking "Is there anything I could be doing differently (or anything I should stop doing) to be more helpful to you/ your child?" Unassertive children or parents may be reluctant to complain, but complaints are often needed to start a fruitful discussion and are preferable to having children drop out of treatment. When talking to children alone, I often ask the follow-up question "Is there anything your parents could be doing differently (or anything they should stop doing) to be more helpful to you?" The answer to this question often reveals important family dynamics that must be incorporated into the formulation and also addressed in treatment. Eliciting parental complaints about the child less often reveals new information, but listening to such complaints may strengthen the therapeutic relationship with the parents, who may feel that their worries and frustrations have not been sufficiently understood.

It is also worth noting that worsening in therapy does not always mean that the formulation was wrong. For example, in anxious children undergoing CBT, the emphasis on feeling identification early in treatment may result in increased anxiety symptoms at that time. In all psychotherapies, anxiety about termination of therapy may result in increased symptoms during the final few weeks. These fluctuations in symptom levels are common and can therefore be anticipated and discussed openly with the child and family. Some negative reactions to therapy are uncommon, however, and therefore more difficult to anticipate. For example, a small number of children and adolescents become distressed when doing relaxation exercises, as they may induce physical sensations that are experienced as "weird" or as loss of control of one's body. Some reasons for deterioration cannot be anticipated at all because they require additional information. For example, in some cultures grandparents are given a great deal of respect and influence in the family, and yet may not be included in mental health assessments of children. Parents may not think it is appropriate to include the grandparent in the context of "Western medicine" or may try to hide the assessment from the grandparent, fearing the possible stigma he or she may associate with a mental health problem in the family. Once treatment starts, however, the grandparent may resent being left out and therefore make disparaging remarks or otherwise undermine progress. Finding out about the grandparent's perspective and including him or her in treatment planning can be very valuable in this case. Doing this may not change the formulation, but it can certainly result in a smoother course of treatment.

Case Example: Serena

Some of the above ideas may become clearer when examining a case example. Let's return to the case of Serena, a young girl described in Chapter 4 who had learning difficulties and severely oppositional behavior, and whose family was in the midst of a high-conflict divorce. Suppose that the assessing practitioner elects to focus intervention on reducing parental conflict in Serena's presence and improving the parents' ability to consistently manage her behavior. The goal would be to stabilize Serena's emotional state by increasing stability in her environment. How would the practitioner respond if Serena's behavior fails to improve after a month or two? First, he or she would have to consider possible reasons for treatment failure, assuming that there is truly no improvement in relation to baseline. One possibility is that Serena's parents are not adhering to the intervention, so nothing has changed. Observing parent–child interactions in the office and (if possible) at home might clarify whether or not this is true. Another possibility is that a few weeks of environmental stability cannot undo the effects of 11 years of exposure to chaos. In this case, persisting with the intervention for a longer time may be indicated. Another possibility is that Serena's difficulty with emotion regulation does not relate to her environment, but rather to her own psychopathology. Perhaps the question of a mood disorder (either unipolar or bipolar) is worth revisiting. Finally, it is possible that Serena is coping with an additional stressor that is fueling her misbehavior (e.g., a new problem at school), resulting in a failure to respond to treatment despite her parents' best efforts.

Before assuming that any of these possibilities is correct, the practitioner ought to meet again with Serena and with her parents. This meeting will allow him or her to elicit further information from everyone that relates to the above possibilities and to reexamine Serena's mental status and the parent–child interactions to determine if either has changed over time. If the parents appear to be working together using consistent behavior management strategies (ideally, confirmed by home observations), Serena's mental status hasn't changed, and no new stresses are reported by the child or parents, encouragement and perseverance are indicated. If the parents do not appear to be adhering to treatment, it may be worth seeking additional resources to help this family. For example, some jurisdictions have organizations that specialize in helping families through divorce; in other jurisdictions, it is possible to locate child and youth workers who can coach parents in behavior management strategies in the home. If a new stress has arisen in Serena's life, this issue should be explored, addressed, and incorporated into the case formulation. If Serena shows a change in mental status (e.g., looking very sad rather than angry on interview), additional treatment may be indicated in combination with continued work on behavior management with the parents. Medication and/or individual therapy might be considered, although it would clearly take Serena some time to trust a therapist given her attachment history. Of course, revision of the case formulation will also be needed. It is important to note that whatever change in treatment is pursued, new baseline measures should be done and a time should be set to reassess progress with Serena and her parents.

THE NEED FOR CONSULTATION

Despite their best efforts to devise a coherent formulation and revise it if needed, all practitioners encounter situations that are baffling or leave them feeling "stuck." In these situations, it is usually helpful to consult one or more colleagues about the case. In some work environments, this happens regularly as people work together on multidisciplinary teams or in peer supervision groups. In other work environments, practitioners must seek out colleagues to consult. In both situations, it is important to be open to colleagues' ideas but maintain clarity about who has primary responsibility for the case.

Experience in children's mental health, specialized areas of expertise, and personal blind spots can all result in one practitioner having an easier time formulating a particular case than a colleague might. Experience often comes into play when trying to understand connections among risk factors. Just as an experienced pathologist sees patterns in tissue under the microscope that a novice might miss, so an experienced mental health practitioner may see patterns in a child's development that are not apparent to a recent graduate. Conversely, sometimes having too much experience with a particular case or type of case can adversely affect our thinking. Someone who sees the child or family with "fresh eyes" can then be helpful. For instance, I have seen children who seemed resistant to trying a new behavior, but a consultation with a colleague revealed the need for a change in their psychotropic medication. Similarly, I have referred challenging cases to family therapists only to be told that the family's treatment readiness was low and the child would do better developing personal strengths or supports (e.g., giving a talented athlete a chance to work with a sympathetic coach; having an adolescent join a youth group).

Specialized areas of expertise are relevant when trying to understand specific types of risk and protective factors. Given the pace of progress in mental health research, most practitioners find it difficult to keep up to date with all types of factors (biological, psychological, social, and cultural/spiritual) and so need to consult colleagues in some areas. For example, I often consult colleagues about factors pertaining to genetics or gene–environment interactions because this aspect of biological research is outside my field of expertise. Similarly, when seeking potential protective factors in a case, I often consult colleagues with cultural or spiritual backgrounds similar to those of the client. In aboriginal communities, for example, sweat lodges, spirit guides, medicine wheels, and other traditional forms of healing can often augment and support evidence-based interventions.

Finally, we all have certain blind spots that can interfere with accurate case formulation. Sometimes these are due to personal developmental issues. For example, we may find certain types of clients annoying or frustrating because they remind us of people who treated us poorly in the past, or gravitate toward certain clients because they remind us of people we loved or admired. Termed "countertransference," these blind spots are sometimes amenable to personal psychotherapy, but a few persist in even the most insightful practitioners. Therefore, wise practitioners never lose their willingness to learn and to nurture an ongoing, healthy curiosity about their clients and about the human condition.

References

Achenbach, T. (2012). *Child Behavior Checklist (6–18)*. Burlington, VT: Author.

Adler, A. (1964). *The individual psychology of Alfred Adler*. (H. L. Ansbacher & R. R. Ansbacher, Eds.). New York: Harper Torchbooks.

Adler-Nevo, G., & Manassis, K. (2009). Outcomes for treatment of anxiety in children: A critical review of long-term follow-up studies. *Depression and Anxiety, 26*, 650–660.

American Academy of Pediatrics. (2012). Children, adolescents, and television. Retrieved from *http://pediatrics.aappublications.org/content/107/2/423.full*.

American Psychiatric Association. (2013). *Diagnostic and statistical manual of mental disorders* (5th ed.). Arlington, VA: Author.

Armstrong, K. (1993). *A history of God*. New York: Ballantine Books.

Armstrong, K. (2012). *The charter for compassion*. Retrieved from *www.charter-forcompassion.org*.

Aten, J. D., O'Grady, K. A., & Worthington, Jr., E. L. (Eds.). (2012). *The psychology of religion and spirituality for clinicians: Using research in your practice*. New York: Routledge.

Bagnell, A., & Bostic, J. (2009). School consultation. In B. J. Kaplan & V. A. Sadock (Eds.), *Comprehensive textbook of psychiatry* (9th ed., pp. 3850–3864). Philadelphia: Lippincott, Williams & Wilkins.

Barbosa, J., Manassis, K., & Tannock, R. (2002). Measuring anxiety: Parent–child reporting differences in clinical samples. *Depression and Anxiety, 15*, 61–65.

Bateson, C. D., Schoenrade, P., & Ventis, L. (1993). *Religion and the individual*. New York: Oxford University Press.

Berk, E. L. (2007). Physical and cognitive development in adolescence. In *Development through the lifespan* (4th ed., pp. 128-140). New York: Pearson Education.

Berlin, L., Zeanah, C. H., & Lieberman, A. F. (2008). Prevention and intervention programs for supporting early attachment security. In J. Cassidy & P. R. Shaver (Eds.), *Handbook of attachment: Theory, research, and clinical applications* (2nd ed., pp. 745–761). New York: Guilford Press.

Bernier, A., Carlson, S. M., Deschenes, M., & Matte-Gagne, C. (2012). Social factors in the development of early executive functioning: A closer look at the caregiving environment. *Developmental Science, 15,* 12–24.

Biederman, J., Hirshfeld-Becker, D. R., Rosenbaum, J. F., Herot, C., Friedman, D., Snidman, N., et al. (2001). Further evidence of association between behavioral inhibition and social anxiety in children. *American Journal of Psychiatry, 158,* 1673–1679.

Block, J., Kemp, G., Smith, M., & Segal, J. (2012, November). Children and divorce. Retrieved from *www.helpguide.org/mental/children_divorce.htm.*

Blos, P. (1979). *The adolescent passage: Developmental issues.* New York: International Universities Press.

Bradley, S. J. (2003). *Affect regulation and the development of psychopathology.* New York: Guilford Press.

Brestan, E. V., & Eyberg, S. M. (1998). Effective psychosocial treatments of conduct-disordered children and adolescents: 29 years, 82 studies, and 5,272 kids. *Journal of Clinical Psychology, 27,* 180–189.

Bretherton, I. (1992). The origins of attachment theory: John Bowlby and Mary Ainsworth. *Developmental Psychology, 28,* 759–775.

Bretherton, I., & Munholland, K. A. (1999). Internal working models in attachment relationships: A construct revisited. In J. Cassidy & P. R. Shaver (Eds.), *Handbook of attachment: Theory, research, and clinical applications* (pp. 89–114). New York: Guilford Press

Carter, C. S., Lederhendler, I. I., & Kirkpatrick, B. (Eds.). (1999). *The integrative neurobiology of affiliation.* Cambridge, MA: MIT Press.

Chassin, L., Rogosch, F., & Barrera, M. (1991). Substance use and symptomatology among adolescent children of alcoholics. *Journal of Abnormal Psychology, 100,* 449–463.

Chaudry, N. M., & Davidson, P. W. (2001). Assessment of children with visual impairment or blindness. In R. J. Simeonsson & S. L. Rosenthal (Eds.), *Psychological and developmental assessment: Children with disabilities and chronic conditions* (pp. 255-247). New York: Guilford Press.

Chess, S., & Thomas, A. (1996). *Temperament.* New York: Routledge.

Cicchetti, D. (1990). An historical perspective on the discipline of developmental psychopathology. In J. Rudolf, A. Masten, D. Cicchetti, K. Nuechterlein, & S. Weintraub (Eds.), *Risk and protective factors in the development of psychopathology* (pp. 2–28). New York: Cambridge University Press.

Cicchetti, D., & Rogosch, F. A. (2002). A developmental psychopathology perspective on adolescence. *Journal of Consulting and Clinical Psychology, 70,* 6–20.

Coie, J., Terry, R., Lenox, K., Lochman, J., & Hyman, C. (1995). Childhood peer rejection and aggression as predictors of stable patterns of adolescent disorder. *Development and Psychopathology, 7,* 697–713.

Conners, C. K. (2008). *Conners 3rd Edition.* Toronto: Multi-Health Systems.

Descartes, R. (1984). Meditations on first philosophy. In *The philosophical writings of Descartes* (Vols. I–III; J. Cottingham, R. Stoothoff, & D. Murdoch, Trans.). Cambridge, UK: Cambridge University Press. (Original work published 1641)

DeSocio, J., & Hootman, J. (2004). Children's mental health and school success. *Journal of School Nursing, 20,* 189–196.

Desrosiers, A. (2012). Development of religion and spirituality across the life span. In J. D. Aten, K. A. O'Grady, & E. L. Worthington Jr. (Eds.), *The psychology of religion and spirituality for clinicians: Using research in your practice* pp. 13–37). New York: Routledge.

Dodge, K. A., & Rutter, M. (Eds.). (2011). *Gene–environment interactions in developmental psychopathology.* New York: Guilford Press.

Doidge, N. (2007). *The brain that changes itself.* New York: Viking USA.

Eells, T. D. (Ed.). (2006). *Handbook of psychotherapy case formulation, 2nd Ed.* New York: Guilford Press.

Egliston, K. A., McMahon, C., & Austin, M. P. (2007). Stress in pregnancy and infant HPA axis function: Conceptual and methodological issues relating to the use of salivary cortisol as an outcome measure. *Psychoneuroendocrinology, 32,* 1–13.

Engel, G. L. (1977). The need for a new medical model: A challenge for biomedicine. *Science, 196,* 129–136.

Englander, E. K. (2012). Spinning our wheels: Improving our ability to respond to bullying and cyberbullying. *Child and Adolescent Psychiatric Clinics of North America, 21,* 43–55.

Erikson, E. H. (1959). *Identity and the life cycle.* New York: International Universities Press.

Faber, A., & Mazlish, E. (2005). *How to talk so teens will listen and listen so teens will talk.* New York: HarperCollins.

Fan, Y., Fike, J. R., Weinstein, P. R., Liu, J., & Liu, Z. (2007). Environmental enrichment enhances neurogenesis and improves functional outcome after cranial irradiation. *European Journal of Neuroscience, 25,* 38–46.

Fox, N. A., & Hane, A. A. (2008). Studying the biology of human attachment. In J. Cassidy & P. R. Shaver (Eds.), *Handbook of attachment: Theory, research, and clinical applications* (2nd ed., pp. 217–240). New York: Guilford Press.

Fowler, J. W. (1981). *Stages of faith.* San Francisco: Harper & Row.

Freud, S. (1933). *New introductory lectures on psychoanalysis.* New York: Penguin Freud Library.

Giardino, J., Gonzalez, A., Steiner, M., & Fleming, A. S. (2008). Effects of motherhood on physiological and subjective responses to infant cries in teenage mothers: A comparison with non-mothers and adult mothers. *Hormones and Behavior, 53*(1), 149–158.

Gonzalez, A., Jenkins, J. M., Steiner, M., & Fleming, A. S. (2012). Maternal early life experiences and parenting: The mediating role of cortisol and executive function. *Journal of the American Academy of Child and Adolescent Psychiatry, 51,* 673–682.

Greene, R. W. (2010). *The explosive child: A new approach for understanding and parenting easily frustrated, chronically inflexible children.* New York: HarperCollins.

Grollman, E. A. (2011). *Talking about death: A dialogue between parent and child.* New York: Beacon Press.

Hanson, J. L., Chung, M. K., Avants, B. B., Rudolph, K. D., Shirtcliff, E. A., Gee, J. C., et al. (2012). Structural variations in prefrontal cortex mediate the relationship between early childhood stress and spatial working memory. *Journal of Neuroscience, 32,* 7917–7925.

Harter, S. (2006). The self. In W. Damon (Series Ed.) & N. Eisenberg (Vol. Ed.), *Handbook of child psychology: Vol. 3. Social, emotional, and personality development* (6th ed., pp. 505-570). New York: Wiley.

Hattie, J. (2009). *Visible learning: A synthesis of over 800 meta-analyses relating to achievement.* New York: Routledge.

Hazan, C., & Shaver, P. R. (1987). Romantic love conceptualized as an attachment process. *Journal of Personality and Social Psychology, 52,* 511–524.

Hoeve, M., Blokland, A., Dubas, J. S., Loeber, R., Gerris, J. R. M., & van der Laan, P. H. (2008). Trajectories of delinquency and parenting styles. *Journal of Abnormal Child Psychology, 36,* 223–235.

Hospital for Sick Children. (2012). Motherisk. Retrieved from *www.motherisk. org/prof/index.jsp.*

Hudson, J. L., & Rapee, R. M. (2001). Parent–child interactions and the anxiety disorders: An observational analysis. *Behaviour Research and Therapy, 39,* 1411–1427.

Ialongo, N., Edelsohn, G., Werthamer-Larsson, L., Crockett, L., & Kellam, S. (1995). The significance of self-reported anxious symptoms in first grade children: Prediction to anxious symptoms and adaptive functioning in fifth grade. *Journal of Child Psychology and Psychiatry, 36,* 427–437.

Kazdin, A. E. (1994). Methodology, design and evaluation in psychotherapy research. In A. E. Bergin & S. L. Garfield (Eds.), *Handbook of psychotherapy and behavior change* (4th ed., pp. 19–71). New York: Wiley.

Kendler, K. S., & Eaves, L. J. (2005). *Psychiatric genetics.* Washington, DC: American Psychiatric Press.

Kirkpatrick, L. A. (1998). God as a substitute attachment figure: A longitudinal study of adult attachment style and religious change in college students. *Personality and Social Psychology Bulletin, 24,* 961–973.

Kovacs, M. (2004). *Children's depression inventory 2.* Toronto: Multi-Health Systems.

Kuyken, W., Padesky, C. A., & Dudley, R. (2009). *Collaborative case conceptualization: Working effectively with clients in cognitive-behavioral therapy.* New York: Guilford Press.

Lazarus, R. S., & Folkman, S. (1984). *Stress, appraisal, and coping*. New York: Springer.

Lewis, H. B. (1971). *Shame and guilt in neurosis*. New York: International Universities Press.

Lieberman, A. F., & Van Horn, P. (2008). *Psychotherapy with infants and young children: Repairing the effects of stress and trauma on early attachment*. New York: Guilford Press.

Magaro, M. M., & Weisz, J. R. (2006). Perceived control mediates the relation between parental rejection and youth depression. *Journal of Abnormal Child Psychology, 34,* 867–876.

Manassis, K. (1986). The effects of cultural differences on the physician–patient relationship. *Canadian Family Physician, 32,* 383–389.

Manassis, K. (2009a). *Cognitive behavioral therapy with children: A guide for the community practitioner*. New York: Routledge.

Manassis, K. (2009b). Silent suffering: Understanding and treating children with selective mutism. *Expert Review in Neurotherapeutics, 9,* 235–243.

Manassis K. (2012). Generalized anxiety disorder in the classroom. *Child and Adolescent Psychiatric Clinics of North America, 21,* 93–103.

Manassis, K., & Kalman, E. (1990). Anorexia resulting from fear of vomiting in four adolescent girls. *Canadian Journal of Psychiatry, 35,* 548–550.

Manassis, K., Wilansky-Traynor, P., Farzan, N., Kleiman, V., Parker, K., & Sanford, M. (2010). The Feelings Club: A randomized controlled trial of school-based intervention for anxious and depressed children. *Depression and Anxiety, 27,* 945–952.

March, J. S. (2004). *Multidimensional anxiety scale for children*. Toronto: Multi-Health Systems.

Marcia, J. E. (1966). Development and validation of ego identity status. *Journal of Personality and Social Psychology, 3,* 551–558.

Masten, A. S., & Coatsworth, J. D. (1998). The development of competence in favorable and unfavorable environments: Lessons from research on successful children. *American Psychologist, 53,* 205–220.

McCue, K. (1996). *How to help children through a parent's serious illness*. New York: St. Martin's Press.

Miller, W. R., & Rollnick, S. (2013). *Motivational interviewing: Helping people change* (3rd ed.). New York: Guilford Press.

Mills-Koonce, W. R., Propper, C., Gariepy, J. L., Barnett, M., Moore, G. A., Calkins, S., et al. (2009). Psychophysiological correlates of parenting behavior in mothers of young children. *Developmental Psychobiology, 51*(8), 650–661.

Monga, S., & Manassis, K. (2006). Treating childhood anxiety in the presence of life-threatening anaphylactic conditions. *Journal of the American Academy of Child and Adolescent Psychiatry, 45,* 1007–1010.

Nelson, J. (2011). What is a hospitalist? *The Hospitalist, 2,* 1.

Newcomb, A. F., & Bagwell, C. L. (1995). Children's friendship relations: A meta-analytic review. *Psychological Bulletin, 117,* 306–347.

Nhat Hanh, T. (1998). *The heart of the Buddha's teaching*. New York: Broadway Books.

Pargament, K. I., Koenig, H. G., & Perez, L. M. (2000). The many methods of religious coping: Development and initial validation of the RCOPE. *Journal of Clinical Psychology, 56*, 519–543.

Parker, J. G., & Asher, S. R. (1993). Friendship and friendship quality in middle childhood: Links with peer group acceptance and feelings of loneliness and social dissatisfaction. *Developmental Psychology, 29*, 611–621.

Parry, G., Roth., A., & Fonagy, P. (2005). Psychotherapy research, health policy, and service provision. In A. Roth & P. Fonagy, *What works for whom?: A critical review of psychotherapy research* (2nd ed., pp. 43–65). New York: Guilford Press.

Pepler, D. J., Jiang, D., & Craig, W. M. (2008). Developmental trajectories of bullying and associated factors. *Child Development, 79*, 325–338.

Persons, J. B. (2008). *The case formulation approach to cognitive-behavior therapy*. New York: Guilford Press.

Piaget, J. (1977). *The essential Piaget*. (H. E. Gruber & J. J. Vonèche, Eds.). New York: Basic Books.

Rapee, R. M., & Melville, L. F. (1997). Recall of family factors in social phobia and panic disorder: Comparison of mother and offspring reports. *Depression and Anxiety, 5*, 7–11.

Reynhout, G., & Carter, M. (2006). Social stories for children with disabilities. *Journal of Autism and Developmental Disorders, 36*, 445–469.

Romans, S. E., & Seeman, M. V. (2006). *Women's mental health: A life cycle approach*. Philadelphia: Lippincott, Williams & Wilkins.

Roth, A., & Fonagy, P. (2005). *What works for whom?: A critical review of psychotherapy research* (2nd ed.). New York: Guilford Press.

Rutter, M. (1995). Clinical implications of attachment concepts: Retrospect and prospect. *Journal of Child Psychology and Psychiatry, 36*, 549–571.

Rutter, M., Bishop, D., Pine, D. S., Scott, S., Stevenson, E. A., & Taylor, A. T., et al. (2010). *Rutter's child and adolescent psychiatry, 5th Ed.* London: Wiley-Blackwell.

Saint-Laurent, G. E. (2011). *Spirituality and world religions: A comparative introduction*. New York: Mayfield.

Seligman, M. E. P., & Csikszentmihalyi, M. (2000). Positive psychology: An introduction. *American Psychologist, 55*, 5–14.

Simeonsson, R. J., & Rosenthal, S. L. (Eds.). (2001). *Psychological and developmental assessment: Children with disabilities and chronic conditions*. New York: Guilford Press.

Skinner, H. A., Steinhauer, P. D., & Santa Barbara, J. (1983). The family assessment measure. *Canadian Journal of Community Mental Health, 2*, 91–105.

Skinner, W. (2009). Approaching concurrent disorders. In *Treating concurrent disorders: A guide for counsellors* (pp. xi–xvii). Toronto: Centre for Addiction & Mental Health.

Skuse, D., & Seigal, A. (2010). Behavioral phenotypes and chromosomal disorders. In M. Rutter, D. Bishop, D. Pine, S. Scott, J. S. Stevenson, E. A. Taylor, et al. (Eds.), *Rutter's child and adolescent psychiatry* (5th ed., pp. 205-240). New York: Wiley-Blackwell.

Spady, D. W., Schopflocher, D. P., Svenson, L. W., & Thompson, A. H. (2001). Prevalence of mental disorders in children living in Alberta, Canada, as determined from physician billing data. *Archives of Pediatric and Adolescent Medicine, 155,* 1153–1159.

Spitz, R. A. (1945). Hospitalism: An inquiry into the genesis of psychiatric conditions in early childhood. *The Psychoanalytic Study of the Child, 1,* 53–74.

Stirling, J. (2007). Beyond Munchausen syndrome by proxy: Identification and treatment of child abuse in a medical setting. *Pediatrics, 119,* 1026–1030.

Stronski, H. S. M., & Remafedi, G. (1998). Adolescent homosexuality. *Advances in Pediatrics, 45,* 107–144.

Taylor, S. E. (2006). *Health psychology* (6th ed.). New York: McGraw-Hill Education.

Tomb, D. A. (2008). *Psychiatry* (7th ed.). Philadelphia: Lippincott, Williams & Wilkins.

Vaillant, G. E. (1992). *Ego mechanisms of defense: A guide for clinicians and researchers.* Washington, DC: American Psychiatric Press.

Valkenburg, P. M., & Peter, J. (2009). Social consequences of the Internet for adolescents: A decade of research. *Current Directions in Psychological Science, 18,* 1–5.

Vanier, J. (2007). *Our life together.* New York: HarperCollins.

Weisz, J. R., & Kazdin, A. E. (Eds.). (2010). *Evidence-based psychotherapies for children and adolescents* (2nd ed.). New York: Guilford Press.

Wentzel, K. R., Barry, C. M., & Caldwell, K. A. (2004). Friendships in middle school: Influences on motivation and school adjustment. *Journal of Educational Psychology, 96,* 195–203.

Williams, K. C. (1996). Piagetian principles: Simple and effective applications. *Journal of Intellectual Disability Research, 40,* 110–119.

Winnicott, D. W. (1965). Ego distortion in terms of true and false self. In *The maturational process and the facilitating environment: Studies in the theory of emotional development* (p. 140–152). New York: International Universities Press.

Wolf, A. E. (2002). *Get out of my life, but first could you drive me and Cheryl to the mall: A parent's guide to the new teenager* (Rev. ed.). New York: Farrar, Straus & Giroux.

World Health Organization. (1994). *International classification of diseases* (10th ed.). Geneva: Author.

Zucker, K. J., & Bradley, S. J. (1995). *Gender identity disorder and psychosexual problems in children and adolescents.* New York: Guilford Press.

Index

Page numbers followed by *t* or *f* indicate tables or figures.